Gynaecological Oncology for the MRCOG and Beyond

Second edition

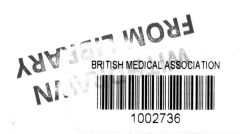

Published titles in the MRCOG and Beyond series

Antenatal Disorders for the MRCOG and Beyond
by Andrew Thomson and Ian Greer

Fetal Medicine for the MRCOG and Beyond
by Alan Cameron, Lena Macara, Janet Brennand and Peter Milton

Gynaecological and Obstetric Pathology for the MRCOG, second edition,
*edited by Michael Wells, C Hilary Buckley and Harold Fox, with a chapter on
Cervical Cytology by John Smith*

Gynaecological Urology for the MRCOG and Beyond
by Simon Jackson, Meghana Pandit and Alexandra Blackwell

Haemorrhage and Thrombosis for the MRCOG and Beyond
edited by Anne Harper

Intrapartum Care for the MRCOG and Beyond
*by Thomas F Baskett and Sabaratnam Arulkumaran, with a chapter on Neonatal
Resuscitation by John McIntyre and a chapter on Perinatal Loss by Carolyn Basak*

Management of Infertility for the MRCOG and Beyond, second edition,
edited by Siladitya Bhattacharya and Mark Hamilton

Medical Genetics for the MRCOG and Beyond
by Michael Connor

Menopause for the MRCOG and Beyond, second edition,
by Margaret Rees

Menstrual Problems for the MRCOG
by Mary Ann Lumsden, Jane Norman and Hilary Critchley

Neonatology for the MRCOG *by Peter Dear and Simon Newell*

Paediatric and Adolescent Gynaecology for the MRCOG and Beyond,
second edition, *by Anne Garden, Mary Hernan and Joanne Topping*

Reproductive Endocrinology for the MRCOG and Beyond, second edition,
edited by Adam Balen

The MRCOG: A Guide to the Examination, third edition,
edited by William Ledger

Gynaecological Oncology for the MRCOG and Beyond

Second edition

Edited by Nigel Acheson and David Luesley

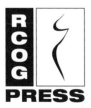

RCOG PRESS

ISBN 978-1-906985-21-9

A machine-readable catalogue record for this publication can be obtained from the British Library [www.bl.uk/catalogue/listings.html]

Published by the **RCOG Press** at the
Royal College of Obstetricians and Gynaecologists
27 Sussex Place, Regent's Park
London NW1 4RG

Registered Charity No. 213280

RCOG Press Editor: Jane Moody
Index: Cath Topliff MA
Design & typesetting: Tony Crowley
Printed in the UK by Latimer Trend & Co. Ltd, Estover Road, Plymouth PL6 7PL

Contents

About the authors   iii

Preface   v

Introduction to the second edition   vii

Abbreviations   viii

1   Basic epidemiology   1
    Andrew Phillips and Nigel Acheson

2   Basic pathology of gynaecological cancer   15
    Raji Ganesan

3   Preinvasive disease of the lower genital tract   35
    Gabrielle Downey

4   Radiological assessment   53
    Sarah Higgins and Adrian Lim

5   Surgical principles   67
    Quentin Davies

6   Role of laparoscopic surgery   85
    Hans Nagar

7   Radiotherapy: principles and applications   95
    David Radstone

8   Chemotherapy: principles and applications   103
    Nigel Acheson

9   Ovarian cancer standards of care   115
    John Kirwan

10   Endometrial cancer standards of care   145
    Rob Gornall

11   Cervical cancer standards of care   155
    Jonathan Herod

12 Vulval cancer standards of care   169
       Michael Hannemann

13 Uncommon gynaecological cancers   189
       Susie Houghton

14 Palliative care   209
       Jo Sykes

15 Emergencies and treatment-related complications   229
       in gynaecological oncology
       Janos Balega and Kavita Singh

Appendix 1: FIGO staging of gynaecological cancers   245

Index   255

About the authors

Nigel Acheson MD FRCOG
Consultant Gynaecological Oncologist,
Royal Devon and Exeter NHS Foundation Trust, Exeter, Devon, UK

Janos Balega MD MRCOG
Consultant Gynaecological Oncologist,
Birmingham Women's Healthcare NHS Trust, City Hospital, Birmingham, UK

Quentin Davies MD FRCS(ED) MRCOG
Consultant Gynaecological Oncologist, Leicester Royal Infirmary, Leicester, UK

Gabrielle Downey MD FRCOG
Consultant Gynaecologist,
Birmingham Women's Healthcare NHS Trust, City Hospital, Birmingham, UK

Raji Ganesan FRCPath
Consultant Histo/Cytopathologist,
Birmingham Women's Healthcare NHS Trust, City Hospital, Birmingham, UK

Robert Gornall FRCS DM MRCOG
Consultant Gynaecological Oncologist, Cheltenham General Hospital,
Cheltenham, UK

Michael Hannemann PhD MRCOG
Consultant Gynaecological Oncologist,
Royal Devon and Exeter NHS Foundation Trust, Exeter, UK

Jonathan Herod MRCOG
Consultant Gynaecological Oncologist,
Liverpool Women's NHS Foundation Trust, Liverpool, UK

Sarah Higgins FRCR
Consultant Radiologist,
South Devon Healthcare NHS Foundation Trust, Torquay, UK

Susie Houghton MRCOG
Consultant Obstetrician and Gynaecologist,
Good Hope Hospital, Sutton Coldfield, UK

John Kirwan MRCOG
Consultant Gynaecological Oncologist,
Liverpool Women's NHS Foundation Trust, Liverpool, UK

Adrian Lim MD FRCOG
Consultant Radiologist,
Imperial College Healthcare Trust, Charing Cross Hospital, London, UK

David M Luesley FRCOG
Professor and Clinical Director for Gynaecology,
City Hospital, Birmingham, UK

Hans Nagar MD MRCOG
Consultant Gynaecological Oncologist,
Belfast City Hospital, Northern Ireland, UK

Andrew Phillips MB ChB MA
Specialist Registrar in Obstetrics and Gynaecology,
Department of Gynaecological Oncology, Centre for Women's Health,
Royal Devon and Exeter NHS Foundation Trust, Exeter, UK

David Radstone DMRT FRCR
Professor of Clinical Oncology, Peninsula Medical School, Exeter, UK

Kavita Singh MD MRCOG
Consultant Gynaecological Oncologist,
Birmingham Women's Healthcare NHS Trust, City Hospital, Birmingham, UK

Joanna Sykes FRCP
Consultant in Palliative Medicine,
South Devon Healthcare NHS Foundation Trust, Torquay, UK

Series editor: Jenny Higham MD FRCOG FFFP ILTM
Consultant Obstetrician and Gynaecologist and Head of Undergraduate
Medicine, Faculty of Medicine, Imperial College London, UK

Preface

Do not be deceived – this volume contains substantial information on a vast subject belying its compact size. Despite the concise nature of the book it does include appropriate subject detail and an acknowledgement of areas of uncertainty. References and data have been updated from the first edition and thus the contemporary information is of great assistance to the potential MRCOG candidate or for those who want to update their knowledge at any career stage. I hope you find this an informative read.

Professor Jenny Higham
Series Editor

Introduction to the second edition

Since the publication of the first edition of Gynaecological Oncology for the MRCOG and Beyond, a multidisciplinary and patient-centred approach to care, delivered in linked local or specialist centres, has been established in the UK. The training of obstetricians and gynaecologists has also changed, with the introduction of advanced training and study modules (ATSM) in the senior years of training. ATSMs in gynaecological oncology and colposcopy can now be undertaken in many centres.

This book will be useful both to those preparing for MRCOG Part 2 and to those undertaking the ATSM in Gynaecological Oncology.

For patients, the pathway of care often begins in local cancer units – this may be confined to diagnosis or may include the triage of patients for further management at a local or specialist centre. This process involves a multidisciplinary approach and usually includes discussion at multidisciplinary team meetings. The contributors to the second edition work as part of such teams throughout the UK.

Recognising these developments in care, the second edition of our book includes chapters which focus on this multidisciplinary approach. We hope that chapters such as those on pathology, radiology, chemotherapy and radiotherapy will increase the understanding of the disciplines that are central to our multidisciplinary teams.

Chapters on laparoscopic surgery, basic surgical principles, palliative care and emergencies and treatment-related complications in gynaecological oncology provide additional up-to-date information for specialists involved in the care of women with gynaecological cancers. The chapters on epidemiology, pathology and each of the main gynaecological cancers have all been updated for this edition and present the latest evidence on investigation, staging and management.

The authors hope that this book will prove to be a valuable resource for those involved in the care of women with gynaecological cancer.

Nigel Acheson
David Luesley
2010

Abbreviations

ACTION	Adjuvant ChemoTherapy In Ovarian Neoplasm trial
AFP	alphafetoprotein
AIS	adenocarcinoma in situ
ASA	American Society of Anesthesiologists
ASTEC	A Study in the Treatment of Endometrial Cancer
AUC	area under the curve
BEP	bleomycin [B], etoposide [E] and cisplatin [P] (chemotherapy regimen)
BIP	bleomycin [B], ifosfamide [I] and cisplatin [P] (chemotherapy regimen)
BMI	body mass index
BRCA1/2	*breast cancer 1/2 gene*
CA125	cancer antigen 125
CAP	cyclophosphamide, doxorubicin and cisplatin (chemotherapy regimen)
CEA	carcinoembryonic antigen
CHORUS	CHemotherapy Or Upfront Surgery trial
CGIN	cervical glandular intraepithelial neoplasia
CIN	cervical intraepithelial neoplasia
CIS	carcinoma in situ
CT	computed tomography
DPAM	disseminated peritoneal adenomucinosis
EMA-CO	etoposide [E], methotrexate [M], actinomycin D [A], cyclophosphamide [C] and vincristine [O] (chemotherapy regimen)
EORTC	European Organisation for Research and Treatment of Cancer
FBC	full blood count
FIGO	International Federation of Gynecology and Obstetrics
GFR	glomerular filtration rate
GOG	Gynecologic Oncology Group
GTD	gestational trophoblastic disease
GTT	gestational trophoblastic tumour
Gy	Gray

hCG	human chorionic gonadotrophin
HiSIL	high-grade squamous intraepithelial lesions
HLA	human leucocyte antigen
HNPCC	hereditary non-polyposis colorectal cancer
HPV	human papillomavirus
HRT	hormone replacement therapy
ICON	International Collaborative Ovarian Neoplasm trial
LDH	lactate dehydrogenase
LLETZ	large-loop excision of the transformation zone
LoSIL	low-grade squamous intraepithelial lesions
LVSI	lymphovascular space invasion
MPA	medroxyprogesterone acetate
MRI	magnetic resonance imaging
NACT	neoadjuvant chemotherapy
NACT-S	neoadjuvant chemotherapy followed by surgery
NHSCSP	National Health Service Cervical Screening Programme
NSAIDs	non-steroidal anti-inflammatory drugs
PVB	cisplatin [P], vinblastine [V] and bleomycin [B] (chemotherapy regimen)
PCR	polymerase chain reaction
PET	positron emission tomography
PMCA	peritoneal mucinous carcinomatosis
POMB-ACE	cisplatin, vincristine, methotrexate and bleomycin; and actinomycin D, cyclophosphamide and etoposide (chemotherapy regimen)
PORTEC	Post Operative Radiation Therapy in Endometrial Carcinoma trial
PSTT	placental site trophoblastic tumour
RECIST	Response Evaluation Criteria in Solid Tumours
RMI	risk of malignancy index
SERM	selective estrogen receptor modulator
SMILE	stratified mucinous intraepithelial lesion
TENS	transcutaneous electrical nerve stimulation
UKCTOCS	United Kingdom Collaborative Trial of Ovarian Cancer Screening
UKFOCSS	United Kingdom Familial Ovarian Cancer Screening Study
VAC	vincristine [V], actinomycin D [A] and cyclophosphamide [C] (chemotherapy regimen)
VAIN	vaginal intraepithelial neoplasia
VEGF	vascular endothelial growth factor
VIN	vulval intraepithelial neoplasia
WHO	World Health Organization

1 Basic epidemiology

Introduction

In recent years there has been a focus on the epidemiology of malignant disease, revealing links such as that between cigarette smoking and lung cancer. Epidemiologists are now investigating characteristics of individuals (for example, genetic factors) or their environment (such as infections and drugs) that may play a part in the development of various cancers.

Information from epidemiological studies is helping to clarify the aetiology of gynaecological cancers. For example, the recognition of preinvasive changes in the genital tract has led to the establishment of cervical screening programmes and of the link with human papillomavirus (HPV), as well as an understanding of the role of estrogen in the development of endometrial cancer. This in turn is helping to plan future prevention and treatment strategies. Table 1.1 shows the incidence, mortality and 5-year survival rates for various cancers.

Cervical cancer

Cervical cancer is a potentially preventable disease, yet it is the second most common cancer in women worldwide. In the UK, cervical cancer is the third most common malignancy to affect the genital tract, after ovarian and endometrial cancer.

The incidence of the disease in the UK has started to change. From 1971 to the mid-1980s, the incidence of cervical cancer remained fairly constant

Table 1.1	Tumour incidence, mortality and 5-year survival rates, UK (2007 data from Cancer Research UK)[14]		
Tumour site	New cases (2001–2006 average)	Deaths at 5 years (2006/2007 data)	Overall 5-year survival, 2007 (%)
Cervix	2270	837	63.1
Uterus	5276	1651	75.5
Ovary	5289	4317	38.9

at 14–16/100 000 but, since 1990, the incidence has fallen to just over 10/100 000. By 2006, a total of 2321 cases had been registered, which represents 1.9% of all cancers in women (excluding non-melanoma skin cancer). However, the age-specific incidence has altered differently in the various age groups, with peak incidences of the disease occurring at 30–34 years and 85+ years and significant decreases at 30–34 years and 70–74 years. These age-specific incidence trends suggest a birth cohort effect, with peaks in risk for women born at the end of the 19th century, in the mid-1920s and after 1950. The latest figures from the National Health Service Cervical Screening Programme (NHSCSP) show that, by 2005, the incidence had fallen to 8.4/100 000.

The mortality associated with cervical cancer has fallen over the second half of the last century in the UK. From 1950 to 1987, the mortality rate decreased annually at a rate of 1.5%, from 11.2/100 000 to 6.1/100 000. The rate of decrease then trebled until 1997, by which time the mortality rate was 3.7/100 000, a total of 1150 deaths, which represented 2% of cancer deaths in women and 0.4% of all deaths in women. In a manner similar to that of incidence trends, the mortality trends also show a birth cohort effect. For example, the risk for women born in 1922 compared with the risk for those women born in 1957 is increased 1.5 times. This increased risk for women born after 1935 coincides with liberalised sexual behaviour associated with the 'swinging sixties'.

CERVICAL CANCER AND HUMAN PAPILLOMAVIRUS

The link between HPV and cervical cancer has been conclusively established. Of the 120 plus subtypes of HPV, around 20 have an association with the lower genital tract. Of these, the most important with respect to the risk of developing cervical cancer are HPV-16 and HPV-18.[1] See Chapter 3 for a fuller discussion of HPV.

RISK FACTORS

Oncogenes

Normal cell regulation signals may be altered by oncogenes. Over-expression of certain oncogenes has been described in many cancers and some studies have linked this with the risk of progression from low- to high-grade cervical intraepithelial neoplasia (CIN).[2]

Genotype

The development of neoplasia in response to HPV infection is to a large extent determined by the host's response to that infection. A link has been reported between women who have the human leucocyte antigen (HLA) DQw3 genotype and cervical cancer.[3] It has also been reported that women with cervical cancer who have the HLA B7 genotype have a poorer prognosis compared with other HLA types.[4] These associations probably reflect the different ways in which particular HLA molecules present HPV peptides to the immune system, with some HLA types being more efficient than others.

Smoking

There is strong epidemiological evidence linking smoking with CIN and cervical cancer.[5] The mechanism for this is unclear but it may be related to a direct mutagenic effect upon cervical squamous cells or to a resulting impaired immune response to HPV infection.[6] Products of smoking such as cotinine, nicotine, hydrocarbons and tars have been isolated in cervical mucus. However, virgins who smoke are not at increased risk of developing cervical cancer. So the presence of a chemical carcinogen alone is not sufficient. Another mechanism which may explain the association is the reduced numbers of antigen presenting Langerhans cells in cigarette smokers.[7] Langerhans cells are dendritic cells responsible for antigen presentation to the immune system. Studies have also found that cutting down or stopping smoking is associated with regression of low-grade CIN.[8]

Hormonal contraception

Women taking the contraceptive pill seem to have an increased incidence of cervical cancer[9] and the risk of developing glandular lesions appears even higher.[10] This risk is independent of the increased chance of contracting HPV if barrier contraception is not used. Why should this be the case? Eversion induced by estrogen stimulates metaplasia, which could lead to an increased risk, and there may be a promotion of expression of viral proteins in women on the pill.

A full discussion of preinvasive disease of the cervix and screening as a preventive strategy can be found in Chapter 3.

Dietary factors

Studies suggesting dietary associations are difficult to control for confounding variables. There is, however, some evidence for a protective effect of beta-carotene, vitamin C and folic acid.[11,12]

Endometrial cancer

Endometrial cancer is the most common gynaecological cancer in the UK, principally affecting postmenopausal women. In the UK, there are approximately 5300 cases of endometrial cancer diagnosed each year, with around 1650[13] deaths from the disease each year.[14] While 93% of cases are diagnosed in women aged 50 years or over, the incidence of endometrial cancer in those aged under 35 years is very low. Peak incidence of 76/100 000 occurs in women aged 64–74 years, with a subsequent reduction in incidence in those aged 80 years and above.

Most women with endometrial cancers develop abnormal vaginal bleeding as an early symptom and their tumours are diagnosed while confined to the uterus. Eight to ten percent of women with postmenopausal vaginal bleeding have cancer. Surgical excision by hysterectomy is often sufficient to treat the disease, but radiotherapy is used when the cancer is more advanced. Recent figures for England show that the age-standardised 5-year survival rate is over 70%. Although, as discussed, over 90% of cases are diagnosed in women over the age of 50 years, younger women can develop the disease. In such cases, symptoms such as intermenstrual bleeding may occur and the diagnosis should be excluded in women with the risk factors cited below.

Some of the strongest epidemiological evidence in the field of gynaecological oncology links the effect of estrogen upon the endometrium with the development of endometrial cancer.

RISK FACTORS

Obesity
In women who are obese, circulating estrogen levels are raised by the conversion of androgens in peripheral fat. These androgens, androstenedione and testosterone, are produced by the adrenal glands.

Polycystic ovary syndrome
Women with polycystic ovary syndrome have an increased risk of endometrial cancer. The long, irregular menstrual cycles are associated with anovulation and unopposed estrogen stimulation. This is explained by the fact that since the duration of the luteal phase is relatively constant, prolongation of the follicular phase results in the long cycles.

Parity
Nulliparous women are at increased risk of developing endometrial cancer. The protective effect of pregnancy appears to be greatest following the first pregnancy, with only modest decreases in risk seen with subsequent pregnancies.

Oral contraceptive pill
A protective effect of the oral contraceptive pill against the development of endometrial cancer is supported by robust epidemiological evidence. The protective effect increases with duration of use but appears to persist for 10–15 years after stopping the pill.

Unopposed estrogen hormone replacement therapy

The risk of endometrial hyperplasia and neoplasia following the use of unopposed estrogen in women with an intact uterus has been well known for over 20 years. A large review published in 1995 assessed 30 studies with adequate controls and risk estimates.[15] The summary relative risk was 2.3 (range 2.1–2.5) for unopposed estrogen, rising to 9.5 for 10 or more years of use. Five years after cessation of use the risk remained elevated at 2.3. The accepted practice of adding at least 10 days of progestogen reduces the relative risk to between 1.0 and 1.8. The relative risk of endometrial cancer death is 2.7 for unopposed estrogen. Women with an intact uterus must not be given unopposed estrogen hormone therapy.

Anti-estrogens

Tamoxifen is a selective estrogen receptor modulator (SERM). It is widely used in the treatment of breast cancer because it competes for estrogen receptors in the breast. However, it stimulates ovarian estrogen biosynthesis and elevates plasma estrogen levels. This increases the risk of endometrial cancer. The relative risk for tamoxifen use of over 5 years has been estimated as 2.0. Newer SERMs have been developed in attempts to produce the ideal SERM, which would have no unwanted effects upon estrogen receptors. One of these, raloxifene, has been shown to have anti-estrogenic effects upon both the breast and endometrium. The risk of endometrial stimulation leading to endometrial cancer could therefore be abolished by using these newer SERMs that are currently under evaluation.[16]

Feminising ovarian tumours

Although rare, feminising ovarian tumours are a risk factor for the development of endometrial cancer. The tumour may be benign (thecoma) or malignant (granulosa cell tumour). Such a diagnosis should be borne in mind in women with evidence of estrogenic endometrial stimulation that is otherwise unexplained.

Diabetes and hypertension

Diabetes and hypertension have also been identified as risk factors for endometrial cancer above and beyond their association with obesity and, thus, increased circulating estrogen levels.[17,18]

Endometrial hyperplasia

Just as cervical cancer has been associated with increasing severity of CIN, endometrial hyperplasia is also a recognised premalignant lesion of the uterus. Similar to CIN, the risk of disease progression in endometrial cancer is associated with the presence of cytological atypia. Hyperplasia alone, whether simple or complex, has only a slight increase in the risk of progression to malignant disease. The addition of cytological atypia, now termed endometrial intraepithelial neoplasia, carries the most risk of progression to malignant disease. Of women undergoing hysterectomy for endometrial intraepithelial neoplasia, 50% will have endometrial cancer diagnosed on pathology specimens.[17]

Ovarian cancer

Ovarian cancer is the fifth most common cancer in women and now has a similar incidence to that of endometrial cancer. In the UK, there are nearly 5300 cases of ovarian cancer diagnosed each year, with around 4300 deaths from the disease each year.[19] It is the most common cause of gynaecological cancer death and affects approximately one in 70 women, with 80% of new cases occurring in women aged over 50 years. This figure exceeds the number of women dying from cervical and endometrial cancers combined. According to data from the International Federation of Gynecology and Obstetrics, 5-year all-stage survival has increased from 27% in the early 1960s to 41% in 2000–2001. Unfortunately, although these data are encouraging, the silent nature of this disease results in 80% having extra-ovarian spread at the time of diagnosis (FIGO stage III or IV) (Table 1.2).

Epidemiological studies have shown that pregnancy, breastfeeding and oral contraceptive use appear to be protective against the development of ovarian cancer. These observations led to the incessant ovulation theory as a possible mechanism of oncogenesis. The basis of this theory is that the repeated mesothelial damage brought about by ovulation results in an increased possibility of a defect in the repair mechanism and eventually malignant transformation. Although superficially attractive, the reduction in incidence seen with just one pregnancy, a short exposure to combined oral contraception and the reduction in incidence occurring after hysterectomy with ovarian conservation have led many to doubt this hypothesis.

Table 1.2	Five-year survival of ovarian cancer for FIGO stages
FIGO stage	5-year survival (from published ranges) (%)
I	71–91
II	38–75
III	16–46
IV	15–21

RISK FACTORS

Parity

Ovarian cancer is more common in nulliparous women and those of low parity. Initial cohort analyses in England and Wales, the USA and Denmark suggested that increased parity was protective. Evidence from subsequent studies confirms that the reduction of ovarian cancer risk is around 10–16% for each pregnancy.[20] To a lesser degree, breastfeeding seems to further reduce the risk of developing ovarian cancer.

Genetic predisposition

Genetic predisposition to epithelial ovarian cancer occurs in up to 10% of women with the disease, but only 7% of women give a family history of ovarian cancer. A familial association in some women with breast and ovarian cancers has been recognised for many years. *BRCA1* and *BRCA2* have been identified as tumour suppressor genes, with mutations being responsible for these familial cases. *BRCA1* is found on chromosome 17 and *BRCA2* on chromosome 13. Those with *BRCA1* mutations have a 40–60% lifetime risk of developing ovarian cancer, while for those with *BRCA2* mutations the risk is lower, at 10–20%. One of the two variants of hereditary non-polyposis colorectal cancer (HNPCC) has also been shown to have an association with ovarian cancer. Known as the Lynch type-II variant of HNPCC, it is associated with a 5–10% lifetime risk of developing ovarian cancer. In addition to the risk of ovarian cancer, women with this variant of HNPCC also have a 30% lifetime risk of developing endometrial cancer.[21]

Discovery of these gene mutations has led to attempts to screen families for the mutations. Currently, over 100 mutations of *BRCA1* have been identified so detecting a mutation in the gene can be difficult. Counselling of those considering such screening must address the difficult issue of managing those in whom a mutation is detected. In young women, future fertility is important and screening, together with estimation of serum CA125 levels and transvaginal ultrasound, may be of benefit and is currently under investigation in a large national trial, the United Kingdom Collaborative Trial of Ovarian Cancer Screening (UKCTOCS). As previously mentioned, there is also evidence to suggest that the oral contraceptive pill may offer some protection to these women.[22] Ultimately, however, prophylactic oophorectomy is likely to provide the greatest benefit. Because ovarian cancers in those with a genetic predisposition occur at an earlier age than sporadic cases, prophylactic surgery is recommended upon completion of a woman's family. It should be noted that in assessing families with a history suggestive of a genetic predisposition, the index case must be shown to carry a genetic mutation, and not to have been a sporadic case.

Oral contraceptive use

Epidemiological studies have shown a significant reduction in ovarian cancer risk in women who have used the combined oral contraceptive pill. With any use, the risk of developing ovarian cancer may be reduced by 36%, with a reduction of up to 70% after 6 years.[22]

For women with a high risk of developing ovarian cancer (such as those with the *BRCA1* or *BRCA2* mutations), studies suggest that this risk can be reduced by 60% by using the combined oral contraceptive pill.[23] There is now a suggestion that the progestogen-only pill may confer an even greater level of protection. The mechanism of action is still somewhat speculative, but progestogens may promote apoptosis in ovarian mesothelium.[24]

Infertility

The possibility of a link between ovulation and ovarian oncogenesis led to concerns that infertility treatments might increase the risk of developing ovarian cancer. This has not been proven.[25] Instead, it seems possible that the slightly increased numbers of cancers observed could be due to the increased risk associated with nulliparity.

Hormone replacement therapy

Those using hormone replacement therapy (HRT) for longer than 5 years have approximately a 20% increase in the risk of ovarian cancer. The risk appears to be bigger in those using estrogen-only HRT relative to estrogen/progesterone therapy. This risk is not apparent in those using HRT for less than 5 years and the risk additionally reduces upon cessation of therapy.[26]

Ovarian irritation

Although the basis of ovarian disease is as yet unproven, evidence has emerged demonstrating an association with perineal talc application and the development of ovarian cancer,[27] the explanation for such a finding being the theory of supposed transmission from the perineum into the abdominal cavity of talc particles leading to irritation of the ovary. Such a theory could explain the reduction in risk of between 18% and 70% noted in those who have undergone tubal ligation. Hysterectomy may additionally reduce the risk of ovarian disease.[28]

Ovarian/peritoneal disease

Those with a hospital diagnosis of ovarian cysts before the age of 29 years have been seen to have an increased risk of ovarian cancer. This risk is increased again in those that additionally have required surgical resection or unilateral oophorectomy. Increased risk as well as an increase in ovarian sited endometrial cancer has been noted in those suffering from endometriosis.[29]

Smoking

Although smoking increases the incidence of mucinous ovarian tumours, it additionally reduces the risk of clear-cell ovarian cancers. Its effect therefore on the risk of ovarian disease overall may be considered equivocal.

Squamous vulval cancer

As for skin cancers elsewhere, 90% of vulval cancers are squamous in origin. The remainder include melanomas, adenocarcinomas and sarcomas. In the UK, there are around 1000 cases of squamous vulval cancer diagnosed each year, with around 350 deaths/year from the disease, resulting in a crude death rate of 1.2/100 000. Apart from its rarity, squamous vulval cancer is a condition that largely affects the elderly: 80% of women with this condition are over 55 years of age. It is not surprising, therefore, that medical comorbidity is high in the vulval cancer population. Such comorbidity poses additional challenges for management and may often influence choices of treatment.

The aetiology is poorly understood but it now seems likely that vulval cancer develops in more than one way. HPVs (HPV16 in particular) have been implicated in the development of vulval intraepithelial neoplasia (VIN) and the subsequent progression to cancer. In addition, women with maturation disorders, such as lichen sclerosus, have an association with invasive vulval carcinoma. Thus, it seems likely that a second mechanism is responsible for malignant transformation. See Chapter 12 for further information on vulval cancer.

RISK FACTORS

Squamous vulval intraepithelial neoplasia

VIN is an uncommon condition and its true incidence is unknown. The incidence of the condition has been thought to be increasing, by up to three-fold.[30,31] Interestingly, the incidence of vulval cancer has remained unchanged. The change in incidence of VIN could be due to an increased awareness of the condition leading to increased detection rates. The increased incidence of VIN is in part due to an increase in the number of young women in whom there appears to be a close association with HPV infection.

The link between HPV, CIN and cervical cancer is well known. The situation is not so clear in women with HPV and VIN. As stated above, the incidence of VIN is increasing, particularly in young women with evidence of HPV infection. The incidence of vulval cancer is not increasing and the majority of women developing cancer at present are older, with VIN not associated with HPV. A small group of women will have several genital tract neoplasias present at the same time, such as VIN, CIN and vaginal intraepithelial neoplasia (VAIN). One study has suggested that such changes are found in up to 25%of women with VIN.[32] These women present a long-term challenge in managing premalignant changes throughout the genital tract.

Beyond HPV infections, it has been noted herpes simplex virus (type 2) antibodies in the blood is, after the presence of HPV has been controlled for, associated with an increased risk of vulval disease.[33] As one would expect, the risk of vulval cancer is also increased in the presence of HIV and medical immunosuppression.

Lichen sclerosus

Lichen sclerosus is an uncommon disease which can affect men and women, with women affected almost six times more commonly than men. Postmenopausal women are the most common group to be affected, although premenopausal women and even young girls can develop the disease. Various aetiological factors have been suggested. Of these, only the link between autoimmune disorders and lichen sclerosus has been clearly demonstrated. One study found that 21.5% of female patients had a history of autoimmune disease, such as thyroid disease, pernicious anaemia and diabetes.[34]

Long-term follow-up is recommended for women with lichen sclerosus. This is based on the risk of malignant transformation, which is thought to be as high as 5% in some series.[35] Some studies have demonstrated an association with psoriasis requiring hospital admission and a threefold increase in the rate of vulval cancer.[36]

Smoking

As discussed, 90% of vulval cancers are squamous in origin and, as such, smoking demonstrates a dose response associated with up to a six-fold increase in vulval disease.[37] Furthermore, infection with HPV16 and a heavy smoking history of greater than 20 cigarettes a day may increase the risk of vulval cancer 25-fold.[38]

KEY POINTS

Cervix

- Increased risk of developing cervical cancer with increasing number of partners.
- Causal link between HPV and cervical cancer.

Endometrium

- Increased risk with obesity, polycystic ovary syndrome, nulliparity, unopposed estrogen hormone replacement therapy, tamoxifen, feminising ovarian tumours.
- Decreased risk with increasing parity, oral contraceptive use.

Ovary

- Decreased risk with parity, breastfeeding, oral contraceptive pill and sterilisation.
- Increased risk with nulliparity (and possibly infertility), genetic predisposition.

Vulva

- Link with both HPV and maturation disorders.

References

1. Schoell WM, Janicek MF, Mirhashemi R. Epidemiology and biology of cervical cancer. *Semin Surg Oncol* 1999;16:203–11.

2. Hayashi Y, Hachisuga T, Iwasaka T, Fukada K, Okuma Y, Yokoyama M, *et al.* Expression of ras oncogene produce and EGF receptor in cervical squamous cell carcinomas and its relationship to lymph node involvement. *Gynecol Oncol* 1991;40:147–51.

3. Wank R, Thomssen C. High risk of squamous cell carcinoma of the cervix for women with HLA-DQw3. *Nature* 1991;352:723–5.

4. Ellis JRM, Keating PJ, Baird J, Hounsell EF, Renouf DV, Rowe M, *et al.* The association of an HPV 16 oncogene variant with HLA-B7 has implications for vaccine design in cervical cancer. *Nat Med* 1995;1:464–70.

5. Trevathan EP, Layde LA, Webster DW, Adams JB, Benigno BB, Ory H. Cigarette smoking and dysplasia and carcinoma-in-situ of the uterine cervix. *JAMA* 1983;250:499–505.

6. Kjellberg L, Hallmans G, Ahren AM, Johansson R, Bergman F, Wadell G, *et al.* Smoking, diet, pregnancy and oral contraceptive use as risk factors for cervical intra-epithelial neoplasia in relation to human papilloma virus infection. *Br J Cancer* 2000;82:1332–8.

7. Barton SE, Jenkins D, Cizick J, Maddox PH, Edwards R, Singer A. Effect of cigarette smoking on cervical epithelial immunity – a mechanism for neoplastic change. *Lancet* 1988;ii:652–4.

8. Szarewski A, Jarvis MJ, Sasieni P, Anderson M, Edwards R, Steele SJ, *et al.* Effect of smoking cessation on cervical lesion size. *Lancet* 1996;347:941–3.

9. Salazar EL, Sojo-Aranda I, Lopez R, Salcedo M. The evidence for an etiologic relationship between oral contraceptive use and dysplastic change in cervical tissue. *Gynecol Endocrinol* 2001;15:23–8.

10. Chilvers C, Mant D, Pike MC. Cervical adenocarcinomas and oral contraceptives. *BMJ* 1987;295:1446–7.

11. Butterworth CE, Hatch K, Macaluso M. Folate deficiency and cervical dysplasia. *JAMA* 1992;267:528–33.

12. Schneider A, Shah K. The role of vitamins in the etiology of cervical neoplasia: an epidemiological review. *Arch Gynecol Obstet* 1989;246:1–13.

13. Cancer Research UK. Uterine cancer: UK uterine (womb) cancer mortality statistics. May 2009 [http://info.cancerresearchuk.org/cancerstats/types/uterus/mortality].

14. London School of Hygiene and Tropical Medicine; National Cancer Intelligence Centre, Office for National Statistics. Cancer survival, England, patients diagnosed 2001–2006 and followed up to 2007: one-year and five-year survival for 21 common cancers, by sex and age. March 2009 [www.statistics.gov.uk/downloads/theme_health/cancer-survival-Eng-2001-2006.pdf].

15. Grady D, Gebretsadik T, Kerlikowske K, Ernster V, Petitti D. Hormone replacement therapy and endometrial cancer risk: a meta-analysis. *Obstet Gynecol* 1995;85:304–13.

16. Dhingra K. Selective estrogen receptor modulation: the search for an ideal hormonal therapy for breast cancer. *Cancer Invest* 2001;19:649–59.

17. Palmer J, Perunovic B, Tidy J. Endometrial hyperplasia. *The Obstetrician & Gynaecologist* 2008;10:211–16.

18. Lucenteforte E, Bosetti C. Diabetes and endometrial cancer: effect modification by body weight, physical activity and hypertension *Br J Cancer* 2007;97:995–8.

19. Cancer Research UK. Ovarian cancer: UK ovarian cancer mortality statistics. May 2009 [http://info.cancerresearchuk.org/cancerstats/types/ovary/mortality].

20. Banks E, Beral V, Reeves G. The epidemiology of epithelial ovarian cancer: a review. *Int J Gynecol Cancer* 1997;7:425–38.

21. Brown GJ, St John DJ, Macrae FA, Aittomaki K. Cancer risk in young women at risk of hereditary nonpolyposis colorectal cancer: implications for gynecologic surveillance. *Gynecol Oncol* 2001;80:346–9.

22. Hankinson SE, Colditz GA, Hunter DJ, Spencer TL, Rosner B, Stampfer MJ. A quantitative assessment of oral contraceptive use and risk of ovarian cancer. *Obstet Gynecol* 1992;80:708–14.

23. Narod SA, Risch H, Moleshi R, Dorum A, Neuhausen S, Olsson H, *et al.* Oral contraceptives and the risk of hereditary ovarian cancer. *N Engl J Med* 1998;339:424–8.

24. Yu S, Lee M, Shin S, Park J. Apoptosis induced by progesterone in human ovarian cancer cell line SNU-840. *J Cell Biochem* 2001;82:445–51.

25. Kashyap S, Moher D, Fung MF, Rosenwaks Z. Assisted reproductive technology and the incidence of ovarian cancer: a meta-analysis. *Obstet Gynecol* 2004;103:785–94.

26. Beral V; Million Women Study Collaborators, Bull D, Green J, Reeves G. Ovarian cancer and hormone replacement therapy in the Million Women Study. *Lancet* 2007;369:1703–10.

27. Merritt MA, Green AC, Nagle CM, Webb PM; Australian Cancer Study (Ovarian Cancer); Australian Ovarian Cancer Study Group. Talcum powder, chronic pelvic inflammation and NSAIDs in relation to risk of epithelial ovarian cancer. *Int J Cancer* 2007;122:170–6.

28. Hankinson SE, Hunter DJ, Colditz GA, Willett WC, Stampfer MJ, Rosner B, *et al.* Tubal ligation, hysterectomy, and risk of ovarian cancer. A prospective study. *JAMA* 1993;270:2813–18.

29. Borgfeldt C, Andolf E. Cancer risk after hospital discharge diagnosis of benign ovarian cysts and endometriosis. *Acta Obstet Gynecol Scand* 2004;83:395–400.

30. Iversen T, Tretli, S. Intra-epithelial and invasive squamous cell neoplasia of the vulva: trends in incidence, recurrence and survival rate in Norway. *Obstet Gynecol* 1998;91:969–72.

31. Sturgeon SR, Brinton LA, Devesa SS, Kurman RJ. In situ and invasive vulvar cancer incidence trends (1973 to 1987). *Am J Obstet Gynecol* 1992;166:1482–5.

32. Shafi MI, Luesley DM, Byrne P, Samra JS, Redman CW, Jordan JA, *et al.* Vulval intra-epithelial neoplasia: management and outcome. *Br J Obstet Gynaecol* 1989;96:1339–44.

33. Sherman KJ, Daling JR, Chu J, Weiss NS, Ashley RL, Corey L. Genital warts, other sexually transmitted diseases, and vulvar cancer. *Epidemiology* 1991;2:257–62.

34. Rowell NR, Goodfield MJD. The connective tissue diseases. In: Champion RM, Burton JL, Burns DA, editors. *Textbook of Dermatology.* Vol. 2. 6th ed. Oxford: Blackwell Science; 1998. p. 2547–53.

35. Meyrick Thomas RH, Ridley CM, McGibbon DH, Black MM. Lichen sclerosus et atrophicus and autoimmunity: a study of 350 women. *Br J Dermatol* 1988;118:41–6.

36. Boffetta P, Gridley G, Lindelöf B. Cancer risk in a population-based cohort of patients hospitalized for psoriasis in Sweden *J Invest Dermatol* 2001;117:1531–7.

37. Daling JR, Sherman KJ, Hislop TG, Maden C, Mandelson MT, Beckmann AM, *et al.* Cigarette smoking and the risk of anogenital cancer. *Am J Epidemiol* 1992;135:180–9.

38. Madeleine MM, Daling JR, Carter JJ, Wipf GC, Schwartz SM, McKnight B, *et al.* Cofactors with human papillomavirus in a population-based study of vulvar cancer. *J Natl Cancer Inst* 1997;89:1516–23.

2 Basic pathology of gynaecological cancer

Introduction

The cellular pathologist plays an important role as a diagnostician and in providing prognostic information by examination of specimens removed for diagnosis and definitive surgery for gynaecological cancers. The pathologist is an essential member of the multidisciplinary team and, through discussion with other team members, helps in formulating important management decisions. This section describes the salient features that would enable the gynaecologist to aid and understand the pathologist in this process.

Sending specimens to the laboratory

FIXATION

Most specimens are sent to the laboratory in fixative, most commonly 10% formalin (4% formaldehyde) solution. Fixation serves to:

- harden tissue to allow sectioning
- preserve tissue by preventing autolysis
- inactivate infectious agents
- enhance avidity for dyes.

The requesting clinician can aid the pathologist by sending the tissue in adequate fixative (10–15 times in volume relative to size of tissue) and by opening large specimens along anatomical planes, thus allowing penetration of fixative.

THE REQUEST FORM

The form accompanying the specimen contains vital details, such as patient details, to prevent misidentification and to prevent serious errors, as well as clinical details, with contact information. Clinical details are important, especially for the pathologist to respond to particular queries. The details should include:

- date and type of procedure
- clinical history, including
  - the purpose of surgery
  - history of prior known disease
  - history of current disease and treatment
  - an indication of urgency of diagnosis
  - menstrual history
  - smear history
  - other relevant details.

FROZEN SECTIONS

Frozen sections are a method of rapidly solidifying small pieces of tissue to make tissue sections for microscopic examination.[1] An intraoperative consultation in gynaecological pathology is indicated:

- to ensure that the tissue sampled is adequate for diagnosis
- to determine the nature of a disease process
- to obtain tissue for research and additional molecular studies
- to determine extent of tumour spread
- to assess the margins.

The information from a frozen section is limited by sampling as only small amounts of tissue can be studied. Challenging situations in intraoperative consultation in gynaecological pathology are:

- diagnosis of malignancy in mucinous tumours
- distinction of an ovarian carcinoma from borderline tumours
- determination of margins in Paget's disease
- distinction between lymphomas and dysgerminoma
- distinction between yolk sac tumour and juvenile granulosa tumour
- lesions biopsied in pregnant women.

Pathology of neoplasia and pre-neoplasia of the female genital tract

CERVIX

Cervical intraepithelial neoplasia

Cervical intraepithelial neoplasia (CIN) is the term used to describe proliferative intraepithelial squamous lesions that display abnormal maturation and cytonuclear atypia. Mitotic activity is often increased and abnormal mitotic forms may be seen. The most important feature is abnormal maturation and this is manifested by loss of polarity and cellular disorganisation. CIN has a three-tier grading system based on the level of involvement of the squamous epithelium by the abnormality.[2] For further information on CIN, see Chapter 3.

GRADING SYSTEM FOR CIN

CIN1   Abnormality confined to basal third of epithelium
CIN2   Abnormality up to lower two-thirds of epithelium
CIN3   Abnormality involving superficial third of epithelium

Immature metaplasia and atrophy are benign lesions that are commonly difficult to differentiate from CIN (Figure 2.1).

Cervical glandular intraepithelial neoplasia

Cervical glandular intraepithelial neoplasia (CGIN) is divided into two tiers: high-grade CGIN, a relatively robust histopathological diagnosis with good inter-observer correlation and correlation with biological potential for malignancy, and low-grade CGIN, which is less well understood and may be under-reported (Table 2.1).

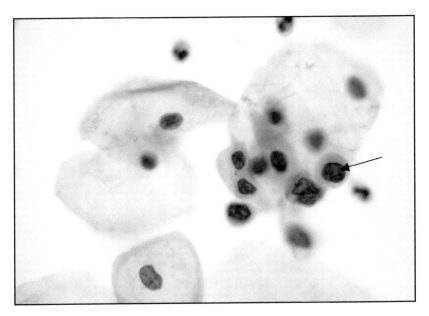

Figure 2.1 This is a dyskaryotic squamous cell (abnormal cell marked with arrow) in a smear taken for screening for cervical cancer. This is indicative of high-grade CIN and the patient will be referred for colposcopy

Table 2.1   Features of high-grade cervical glandular intraepithelial neoplasia

Architectural	Cytological
Gland crowding	Cellular stratification
Branching and budding	Loss of cytoplasmic mucin
Presence of intraluminal papillary projections	Nuclear enlargement Loss of polarity Increased mitotic activity

Distinguishing high-grade CGIN from invasive adenocarcinoma in its earliest stages is difficult and features that raise the possibility of invasion are back-to-back arrangement of glands with little stroma, cribriform gland pattern, desmoplastic stromal response and increased cytoplasmic eosinophilia (Figure 2.2).[3]

Stratified mucinous intraepithelial lesion
Stratified mucinous intraepithelial lesion (SMILE) is a type of intraepithelial neoplasia identified by the presence of conspicuous cytoplasmic

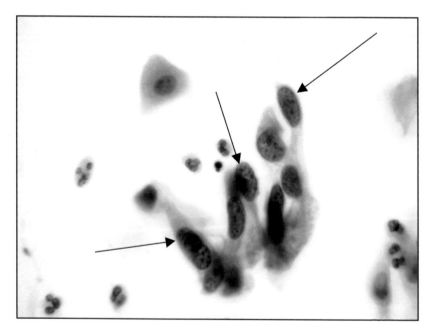

Figure 2.2 A cervical smear showing glandular dyskaryosis (abnormal cells marked with arrows) indicative of high-grade CGIN and the patient will be referred for colposcopy

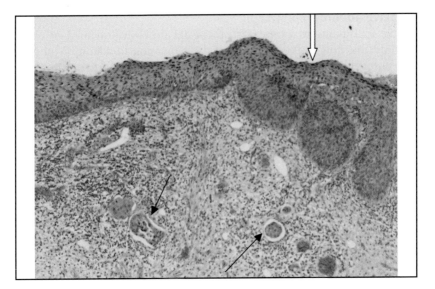

Figure 2.3 This is a tissue section showing CIN3 (block arrow) and small groups of invasive squamous carcinoma cells (thin arrows) in vascular spaces; stromal invasion was present elsewhere in the specimen

vacuoles in lesions otherwise resembling CIN.[4] It is believed to be a variant of glandular intraepithelial neoplasia and may be associated with adenosquamous carcinomas.

Invasive squamous carcinoma

A simple two-tiered classification is recommended and this is based on whether the cells show keratin production and thus are keratinising or lack of keratin production and therefore are non-keratinising. This avoids nosological confusion with small-cell carcinoma, a term that is reserved for tumours showing neuroendocrine differentiation and poorer outcome. Tumour type, presence of vascular invasion and depth of invasion (stage of disease) are the main pathological prognosticators. Histological grade does not appear to have a major influence on outcome (Figure 2.3).

FIGO STAGE IA CARCINOMA

- Maximum size: 5 mm deep and 7 mm in horizontal dimension
- Stage IA1: maximum depth of invasion 3 mm
- Stage IA2: maximum depth of invasion 5 mm
- Vascular space involvement does not affect staging

Invasive adenocarcinoma

Unlike its squamous counterpart, there are no clearly defined or easily reproducible criteria for diagnosis of early invasion in adenocarcinomas. The outcome in these cancers depends upon size, stage and grade. There are several different histological subtypes. There may be difficulties in differentiating an endometrioid variant from a uterine primary and immunohistochemistry may be helpful.[5]

Minimum deviation adenocarcinoma (adenoma malignum) is an extremely well-differentiated variant of endocervical adenocarcinoma with the following features:

- little or no cytological atypia
- little mitotic activity
- presence of glands deep within the cervical stroma beyond the normal crypt field
- sometimes vascular and perineural invasion
- a known association with ovarian sex cord stromal tumour with annular tubules (in Peutz–Jeghers syndrome) and mucinous neoplasms.

HISTOLOGICAL MIMICS OF CGIN AND ENDOCERVICAL ADENOCARCINOMA

- Endometriosis
- Tuboendometrioid metaplasia
- Microglandular adenosis
- Hyperplasia of mesonephric remnants
- Arias-Stella reaction involving endocervical glands.

Adenosquamous carcinoma

The adenosquamous carcinoma variant appears more frequently in younger women. The tumours contain malignant squamous and glandular cells and it may also be possible to identify adjacent CIN and CGIN.

ENDOMETRIUM

Endometrial carcinoma

Carcinoma of the endometrium has increased in frequency compared with carcinoma of the cervix. In Western countries, it is now the most common gynaecological cancer. Simplistically and conceptually, there are two types of endometrial carcinomas: type-1, estrogen-related, endometrioid carcinoma and type-2, non-estrogen-related, prototypically serous carcinomas (Table 2.2).[6] The more common type-1 carcinoma has a precursor endometrial hyperplasia. The precursor of type-2 carcinoma is

Table 2.2   Differences between type-1 and type-2 endometrial carcinoma

	Type 1	Type 2
Characteristic		
Prototype morphology	Endometrioid	Serous
Aetiology	Unopposed estrogen	Unknown
Background endometrium	Hyperplastic	Atrophic
Response to hormone therapy	Can be responsive to progesterone	None
Genetic abnormality		
P53 mutation	10–20%	> 90%
K-ras, catenin	15–40%	0–5%
PTEN inactivation	Up to 50%	< 10%
HER2/neu	Not known	18–80%

termed endometrial intraepithelial carcinoma.

Endometrial hyperplasia

Hyperplasia of the endometrium is characterised by an increase in glandular tissue relative to stroma, with concomitant architectural and sometimes cytological abnormalities.[7] The International Society of Gynecological Pathologists and World Health Organization (WHO) have proposed a classification system in which architectural and cytological

Table 2.3   World Health Organization (WHO) classification of hyperplasia of the endometrium

Pattern	Cytological atypia	WHO	Simplified WHO
Rounded glands with regular outlines	None	Simple hyperplasia	Endometrial hyperplasia
Closely packed glands with irregular outlines	None	Complex hyperplasia	Endometrial hyperplasia
Rounded glands with regular outlines	Focal	Simple hyperplasia with atypia	Atypical endometrial hyperplasia
Closely packed glands with irregular outlines	Multifocal or diffuse	Complex hyperplasia with atypia[a]	Atypical endometrial hyperplasia

[a] This pattern has about a 25% risk of progressing to carcinoma

features are independently evaluated (Table 2.3).

Complex hyperplasia with atypia is difficult to separate from well-differentiated endometrial carcinoma. Helpful histological features include a complex cribriform pattern, intraglandular bridging and polymorphs, abnormal mitotic activity and fibroblastic stromal response.

In women who undergo hysterectomy soon after sampling showing complex atypical hyperplasia, an endometrioid carcinoma is seen in 17–45% of cases. When such cancer is discovered, it is almost always a low-grade, low-stage carcinoma.

The diagnosis of endometrial hyperplasia has been shown to be an area of gynaecological pathology with low diagnostic reproducibility. Even after accounting for extrinsic factors such as scanty sample or low volume hyperplasia, there is disagreement among pathologists, both specialist and general, in diagnosis of complex hyperplasia and cytological atypia.

Uterus

MIXED TUMOURS OF THE UTERUS

Mixed tumours of the uterus contain a mixture of glands and mesenchymal tissue: müllerian adenomyomas, including adenomyoma of endocervical type, typical adenomyomas of endometrioid type, atypical polypoid adenomyoma (typically solitary, well-circumscribed, polypoid lesions of reproductive-age women that contain endometrioid glands with varying degrees of architectural and cytological atypia are separated by myofibromatous stroma). On removal, these may recur in up to 45% of cases. In some instances, they are associated with endometrial carcinomas.

Uterine carcinosarcomas (malignant mixed müllerian tumours) are highly aggressive and have traditionally been regarded as a subtype of uterine sarcoma. However, in recent years, convincing evidence has suggested that most, but not all, are monoclonal in origin rather than true collision tumours. Data confirm that the carcinomatous element is the 'driving force' and that the sarcomatous component is derived from the carcinoma or from a stem cell that undergoes divergent differentiation. Thus, uterine carcinosarcomas are best regarded as metaplastic carcinomas.

TUMOURS OF THE UTERINE WALL

Endometrial stromal tumours

Endometrial stromal tumours of the uterus are the second most common mesenchymal tumours of the uterus. According to WHO classification, they are divided into endometrial stromal nodules, low-grade endometrial stromal sarcomas and undifferentiated endometrial sarcomas (Figure 2.4; Table 2.4).

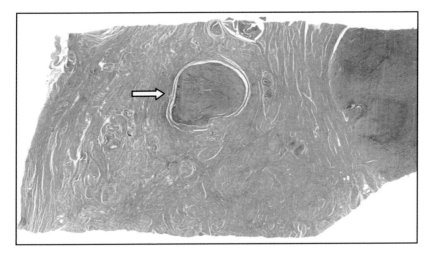

Figure 2.4 The uterine wall show the presence of a low-grade endometrial sarcoma with characteristic permeation of vascular channels (arrow); 4x objective magnification

Smooth muscle tumours of the uterus

The most common tumour of the smooth muscle in the uterus is the benign leiomyoma. Several variants have been described. Smooth muscle tumours of the uterus also include smooth-muscle tumour of unknown malignant potential and leiomyosarcoma.[8] The terminology surrounding these various tumours is shown in Table 2.5.

Ovary

OVARIAN TUMOURS

There are three main groups of primary ovarian tumours: epithelial tumours that are derived from müllerian epithelium; sex-cord or stromal

Table 2.4   Endometrial tumours with a stromal component

Component	Endometrial stromal nodule	Endometrial stromal sarcoma
Non-epithelial	+	+
Epithelial: 　benign 　malignant	– –	– –
Stromal: 　benign 　malignant	+ –	+ (invasive margin) + (invasive margin)

Table 2.5   Smooth muscle tumours of the uterus

Name	Features	Comment
Cellular and highly cellular leiomyoma	Cytologically bland Mitotic activity < 5 MFs/10 HPF	Benign
Leiomyoma with bizarre nuclei	Variable numbers of cytologically bizarre nuclei No CTCN Mitoses < 10 MFs/10 HPF	Benign
Mitotically active leiomyoma	5–15 MFs/10 HPF Commonly submucosal, typically secretory phase due to mitogenic effect of progestins May be associated with use of GnRH agonists	Benign
Leiomyosarcoma	CTCN, diffuse moderate to marked cytological atypia, usually high mitotic rate	Malignant
Myxoid smooth muscle tumour	Myxoid background Difficult to evaluate because of low mitotic activity and focal atypia	Difficult to predict, extensive sampling advised
Atypical leiomyoma	Diffuse significant atypia < 10 MFs/10 HPF No CTCN With higher mitotic activity	Low risk of recurrence, experience limited
Smooth muscle tumour of low malignant potential	CTCN present, no more than mild atypia, less than 10 MFs/10 HPF	Controversial category
Smooth muscle tumour of unknown malignant potential	Other combination of features of concern falling short of leiomyosarcoma	

CTCN = coagulative tumour cell necrosis; HPF = high-power field: MFs = mitotic figures

tumours, derived from the ovarian stroma, sex-cord derivatives or both; and germ cell tumours, which originate from the ovarian germ cells. The most common malignant tumours are serous, mucinous and endometrioid adenocarcinomas. The most common ovarian tumours are:

- mature cystic teratoma (dermoid cyst of the ovary)
- serous cystadenoma
- mucinous cystadenoma
- serous carcinoma

- fibroma-thecoma
- borderline serous tumour
- endometrioid carcinoma
- borderline mucinous tumour
- mucinous carcinoma.

Borderline serous tumours

Borderline serous tumours are characterised by complex branching of papillae either from the cyst lining or on the ovarian surface, cellular proliferation and stratification, variable nuclear atypia and mitotic activity, and clear demarcation from underlying stroma.[9]

- stromal microinvasion

  Focus or foci of destructive stromal invasion measuring less than 3 mm. In the absence of extra-ovarian disease, this does not alter the prognosis. Stromal invasion appears to be more commonly seen in pregnant women.[10]

- implants

  Deposits of tumour in peritoneum or omentum, seen in 15–30% of borderline serous tumours (Table 2.6).

Micropapillary serous carcinoma

Micropapillary serous carcinoma is a histological variant of borderline serous tumour characterised by long, thin papillae seen arising directly from a large papilla. The usual hierarchical pattern in conventional serous tumours is not seen. When florid, it is believed to indicate a prognosis closer to a serous carcinoma, even in the absence of stromal invasion.

OVARIAN CARCINOMA

Subclassification of ovarian carcinomas is biologically and increasingly therapeutically important. The traditional morphologic approach is that the most common type of ovarian carcinoma is the high-grade serous carcinoma. Mucinous carcinomas are uncommon and should only be

Table 2.6 Implants

Type of implant	Appearance	Implication
Non-invasive	Surface growth only	No prognostic significance
Desmoplastic	Desmoplastic response in underlying stroma, no invasion	No prognostic significance
Invasive	Invasion of underlying tissue	Poorer outcome

diagnosed after the possibility of metastatic carcinoma is excluded. True ovarian mucinous carcinomas are usually well-differentiated. They are of two types: intestinal and müllerian mucinous (seromucinous) and they are histogenetically and clinically distinct. Müllerian mucinous carcinomas and clear-cell carcinomas are associated with endometriosis. Ovarian endometrioid carcinomas morphologically resemble endometrioid carcinomas of endometrium.

The pathogenesis of ovarian carcinomas has been widely researched.[11] There is some evidence to support the theory that all serous carcinomas originate in the distal end of the fallopian tube and secondarily spread to the ovary. More recently, surface epithelial tumours have been divided into two broad categories, designated type-I and type-II tumours, that correspond to two main pathways of tumorigenesis. Type-I tumours include low-grade serous carcinoma, mucinous, endometrioid and clear-cell carcinomas. They are genetically stable and are characterised by mutations in a number of different genes, including *KRAS, BRAF, PTEN* and beta-catenin. Type-II tumours are rapidly growing highly aggressive neoplasms, for which well-defined precursor lesions have not been described. Type-II tumours include high-grade serous carcinoma, carcinosarcomas and undifferentiated carcinomas. This group of tumours has a high level of genetic instability and is characterised by mutation of *p53*. This pattern of tumour indicates a poorer prognosis and a poorer response to platinum-based chemotherapy than other morphological types of ovarian cancer.

Vulva

VULVAL INTRAEPITHELIAL NEOPLASIA

The term VIN encompasses a spectrum of intraepidermal pathology of the vulval skin or mucosa, ranging from mild atypia to severe abnormalities amounting to carcinoma in situ. Increasingly, two types of VIN are recognised. The easily diagnosed warty or basaloid VIN occurs in younger women and has an aetiological association with human papillomavirus. The differentiated or simplex VIN is seen in older women and is associated with lichen sclerosis.[12]

Grading system for VIN	
VIN1	Abnormalities confined to basal layers (lower one-third)
VIN2	Dysplastic keratinocytes confined to lower two-thirds.
VIN3	Abnormal cells occupy full thickness of the epithelium

Patterns of VIN

Warty	Presence of multinucleate cells and koilocytes indicative of human papillomavirus
Basaloid	Smaller, more compact. basaloid cells with less pleomorphism and fewer atypical mitoses
Differentiated	Abnormal cells confined to the basal and parabasal layers with keratin pearl formation

SQUAMOUS-CELL CARCINOMA

Squamous-cell carcinoma is an invasive tumour showing squamous differentiation. Superficially invasive squamous carcinoma is a term used when the depth of invasion is ≤ 1 mm. The depth of invasion differs from tumour thickness and is measured from the epithelial stromal junction of the most superficial adjacent normal dermal papilla to the deepest invasive tumour. Tumour thickness is measured from the surface (if ulcerated) or granular layer of overlying keratinised surface to the deepest point of invasion.

VERRUCOUS CARCINOMA

Verrucous carcinoma is a well-differentiated and biologically low-grade neoplasm. To fit into this category, strict histological criteria must be fulfilled. These include pushing borders, no frank destructive invasion and large keratinocytes with pale eosinophilic cytoplasm and sparse mitotic activity.

EXTRAMAMMARY PAGET'S DISEASE

The vulva is one of the most commonly involved sites in extramammary Paget's disease. The origin of this neoplasm is unclear. Histological features are clonal nests or single pale cells in the epidermis; rarely, invasive elements are seen; mucin stains positive.

MELANOMA

Melanoma accounts for about 9% of all malignant vulval tumours. Clark's levels of invasion can be applied to vulval melanomas. Breslow's thickness (in mm) measures the thickness of a melanoma. Poorer outcome is indicated by:

- Breslow's thickness greater than 0.76 mm
- Clark's level greater than II
- Vascular involvement.

PERITONEAL PATHOLOGY

Mesothelial lesions:

- Mesothelial hyperplasia
- Multicystic mesothelioma:
  - occurs predominantly in women of reproductive age
  - involves the pelvic peritoneum
  - may recur after surgical removal
- Well-differentiated papillary mesothelioma:
  - well-developed coarse papillae are seen
  - clinical behaviour is usually prolonged and largely benign
- Malignant mesothelioma:
  - invasive tumour with poor prognosis
  - important for pathologist to distinguish from peritoneal carcinomas

Lesions of the secondary müllerian system:

- Serous lesions:
  - endosalpingiosis
  - peritoneal serous borderline tumours
  - serous psammocarcinoma
  - peritoneal serous carcinoma
- Mucinous lesions:
  - endocervicosis
  - pseudomyxoma peritonei

Mucinous neoplasms involve the peritoneal surfaces and manifest with an extensive collection of mucinous material in the abdomen referred to clinically as pseudomyxoma peritonei or gelatinous ascites.[13] Pathologically, there are fundamentally two main types of mucinous tumours. The low-grade lesions are variably referred to as disseminated peritoneal adenomucinosis (DPAM) and mucinous carcinoma peritonei, low-grade. These tumours typically have a better prognosis. The group that is associated with poor prognosis is designated as peritoneal mucinous carcinomatosis (PMCA), mucinous carcinoma or mucinous carcinoma peritonei, high-grade. Intermediate, mixed, hybrid, or discordant features can be seen. The low-grade lesions are typically associated with an appendiceal tumour and in many cases there is involvement of ovaries that may outsize an unremarkable appearing appendix. In these cases, the cellularity is low and the neoplastic cells are bland. The high-grade lesions show a pattern of spread typical of carcinoma including involvement of lymph nodes and metastasis outside the abdominal cavity. On microscopy, the lesions are more cellular and the cells show obvious features of malignancy. The primary tumour is generally from the gastrointestinal tract.

Special studies in pathology

The haematoxylin and eosin stain is the basic stain used primarily on every specimen by a pathologist. Familiarity with the special studies available is important for the clinician because the initial handling of the specimen may limit the types of studies that can be performed.

HISTOCHEMISTRY

All histochemical stains can be performed on formalin-based tissue. Table 2.7 shows the commonly used stains and their possible applications.

IMMUNOHISTOCHEMISTRY AS A DIAGNOSTIC TOOL

Immunohistochemistry or immunocytochemistry is a diagnostic tool used by cellular pathologists for accumulating evidence to support a diagnostic possibility after the conventional stains have generated a differential diagnosis. This technique localises target antigens on cells with the help of antigen-specific antibodies (primary antibodies) applied to formalin-fixed,

Table 2.7	Commonly used stains and their possible applications	
Stain	Components stained	Comments
Periodic acid – Schiff stain (PAS)	Glycogen, neutral mucin	Highlights glycogen and mucin in cells
PAS with diastase digestion	Mucin	Glycogen is digested by diastase and therefore not stained
Alcian blue	Acid mucins	Can identify intestinal type mucin
Ziehl–Nielsen stain	Mycobacteria	To identify tuberculosis bacillus
Toluidine blue	Mast cells	

Table 2.8   Commonly used antibodies and their significance

Antibody	Tissue identified
Cytokeratin	Epithelial
S100	Neural, melanocytic
HMB45	Melanocytic
Vimentin	Mesenchymal
Inhibin	Sex-cord elements
CA125	Mesothelial/müllerian
Leucocyte common antigen	Leucocytes
CD10	Endometrial stroma
Human chorionic gonadotrophin	Trophoblast
Human placental lactogen	Trophoblast
Placental alkaline phosphatase	Germ cell elements
Alphafetoprotein	Yolk sac elements
Smooth muscle antigen, desmin	Smooth muscle
Chromogranin	Neuroendocrine
Thyroglobulin	Thyroid

paraffin-embedded tissue sections. A secondary antibody-based reagent is then used to colour the target molecule at the specific interaction site. The specificity and sensitivity of the primary antibody, the presence of the antibody at the specific site and the perfection of techniques of antigen retrieval are important in interpretation of the results. Commonly used antibodies and their significance are shown in Table 2.8. The major role of immunohistochemistry in diagnostic gynaecological pathology is in differentiating between primary and metastatic carcinoma of the ovary.[14]

Metastatic carcinomas to the ovary account for up to 7% of all ovarian neoplasms. Primary endometrioid carcinoma is closely mimicked by a metastatic colonic carcinoma. Differential staining with cytokeratin 7 (CK7) and CK20 can be used to separate these histologically similar entities (Table 2.9). Evaluation of metastatic carcinoma should include:

Table 2.9   Differential staining to separate histologically similar entities

CK20	CK7 positive	CK7 negative
Positive	Urothelial carcinomas Pancreaticobilary carcinomas Mucinous ovarian neoplasms	Colorectal carcinomas
Negative	Breast carcinoma Non-mucinous ovarian carcinomas	Hepatocellular carcinomas Renal cell carcinomas

CK = cytokeratin

Table 2.10 Paget's disease versus superficially spreading melanoma				
	S100	*HMB45*	*CAM5.2*	*EMA*
Paget's disease	–	–	+	+
Superficial spreading	+	+	–	–
EMA = epithelial membrane antigen				

- morphology
- clinical history
- operative findings: extra-ovarian tumour
- histology: bilaterality, surface tumour, multi-nodularity, vascular invasion
- clinical relevance of determining primary site
- immunohistochemical panel (Table 2.9).

Extramammary Paget's disease
Table 2.10 distinguishes extramammary Paget's disease from superficially spreading melanoma.

Evaluating spindle tumours of the myometrium
Table 2.11 differentiates endometrial stromal from smooth muscle tumours.

Glandular lesions of the cervix
These immunohistochemical stains are discriminatory in many cases (Table 2.12).

Peritoneal mesothelioma and serous carcinoma in the peritoneum
Peritoneal mesothelioma and serous carcinoma in the peritoneum are difficult to distinguish histologically and, when there is diffuse involvement, immunohistochemistry can be of considerable ancillary value. In the differentiation between papillary serous carcinoma of the peritoneum and serous carcinoma of the ovary, immunohistochemical studies are of limited value as they have a similar phenotype.

Table 2.11 Endometrial stromal versus smooth muscle tumours					
	CD10	*CD34*	*SMA*	*Desmin*	*h-caldesmin*
Endometrial stromal tumours	+	–	-	+ Focal	–
Smooth muscle tumours	+	±	+	+ Diffuse	+
SMA = smooth muscle antigen					

Table 2.12 Glandular lesions of the cervix

	CEA	HMFG1	EMA	CD44v5
Normal epithelium	+\–ve/luminal+ve	+\–ve/luminal+ve	–ve/basolateral+ve	+ve
CGIN	cytoplasmic+ve	cytoplasmic+ve	+ Diffuse	–ve

CGIN = cervical glandular intraepithelial neoplasia; CEA = carcinoembryonic antigen; EMA = epithelial membrane antigen; HMFG1 = human milk fat globulin 1

PROGNOSTIC VALUE OF IMMUNOHISTOCHEMICAL MARKERS

Cancer prognosis has always been based on histological typing and grading, imaging findings and clinical stage of patients. While this is valid in population or group-based studies, it is of little relevance to the individual patient or tumour. Immunohistochemistry is now being used both at research and practice levels to identify subsets of patients who will be likely to benefit from additional therapy. Not all the methods listed below are in use for gynaecological tumours but the list provides some indication of what lies ahead in the field of gynaecological oncology.

Tumour microstaging
The following will help to accurately stage tumours by detecting micrometastases or vascular invasion, thus aiding appropriate treatment:

- detection of microinvasion by use of quantitative and qualitative assessment of immunohistochemistry for basement membranes
- use of vascular markers (factor VIII-related protein, CD31, CD34) to detect vascular space involvement.

Markers to predict response to therapy
Estrogen and progesterone receptors in breast cancer provide information for prognostication, as well as helping to inform decisions regarding hormonal manipulation of the tumour. Steroid-regulated proteins cathepsin D and pS2 serve as post-receptor markers for a functional estrogen receptor pathway.

C-erbB-2 gene alterations have been reported in many tumours. In breast cancer, c-erbB-2 positive tumours can be treated with the anti-c-erbB-2 drug herceptin. Others include:

- tumour suppressor genes
- tumour angiogenesis
- anti-apoptosis genes

- DNA repair genes
- adhesion molecules.

Molecular pathology

Molecular pathology incorporates many techniques in use for the investigation of genetic alterations in cells and organisms. Techniques include polymerase chain reaction (PCR), Southern blotting and in situ hybridisation. Molecular genetic pathology has application in three main areas: identification of inherited diseases, detection of microorganisms and, in cancer, identification of specific genetic alterations, identification of clonality and detection of minimal residual disease.

References

1. Baker P, Oliva E. A practical approach to intraoperative consultation in gynaecological pathology. *Int J Gynecol Pathol* 2008;27:353–65.

2. Buckley CH, Butler EB, Fox H. Cervical intraepithelial neoplasia. *J Clin Pathol* 1982;35:1–13.

3. El-Ghobashy AA, Shaaban AM, Herod J, Herrington CS. The pathology and management of endocervical glandular neoplasia. *Int J Gynecol Cancer* 2005;15:583–92.

4. Park JJ, Sun D, Quade BJ, Flynn C, Sheets EE, Yang A, *et al*. Stratified mucin-producing intraepithelial lesions of the cervix: adenosquamous or columnar cell neoplasia? *Am J Surg Pathol* 2000;24:1414–19.

5. Hart WR. Symposium Part II: Special types of adenocarcinoma of the uterine cervix. *Int J Gynecol Pathol* 2002;21:327–46.

6. Prat J, Gallardo A, Cuatrecasas M, Catasus L. Endometrial carcinoma: pathology and genetics. *Pathology* 2007;39:72–87.

7. Clement PB, Scully RE. Endometrial hyperplasia and carcinoma. In: Clement PB, Young RH, editors. *Tumors and Tumorlike Lesions of the Uterine Corpus and Cervix*. New York: Churchill Livingstone; 1993. p. 85–136.

8. Toledo G, Oliva E. Smooth muscle tumors of the uterus: a practical approach. *Arch Pathol Lab Med* 2008;132:595–605.

9. Bell DA, Longacre TA, Prat J, Kohn EC, Soslow RA, Ellenson LH, *et al*. Serous borderline (low malignant potential, atypical proliferative) ovarian tumours: workshop perspectives. *Hum Pathol* 2004;35;934–48.

10. Mooney J, Silva E, Tornos C, Gershenson D. Unusual features of serous neoplasms of low malignant potential during pregnancy. *Gynecol Oncol* 1997;65:30–5.

11. Kurman RJ, Shih I. Pathogenesis of ovarian cancer: lessons from morphology and molecular biology and their clinical implications. *Int J Gynecol Pathol* 2008;27:151–60.

12. Hart WR. Vulvar intraepithelial neoplasia: historical aspects and current status. *Int J Gynecol Pathol* 2001;20:16–30.

13. Ronnett BM, Kurman RJ, Zahn CM, Shmookler BM, Jablonski KA, Kass ME, *et al*. Pseudomyxoma peritonei in women: a clinicopathologic analysis of 30 cases with emphasis on site of origin, prognosis, and relationship to ovarian mucinous tumors of low malignant potential. *Hum Pathol* 1995;26:509–24.

14. Yaziji H, Gown AM. Immunohistochemical analysis of gynaecologic tumors. *Int J Gynecol Pathol* 2001;20:64–78.

3 Preinvasive disease of the lower genital tract

Introduction

This chapter concentrates mainly on premalignancy of the cervix, as this is the most common of the preinvasive conditions and the only one that is screened for on a population basis. Most of the information about cervical premalignancy refers to squamous lesions, as these are by far the most frequent. Preinvasive disease of the glandular endocervical epithelium will also be considered, as will preinvasive conditions of the vagina and vulva.

Preinvasive disease and terminology

The concept of precancer of the cervix dates back to the end of the 19th century, when Sir John Williams described non-invasive tissue resembling malignancy adjacent to an area of microinvasive carcinoma in a hysterectomy specimen. The term carcinoma in situ (CIS) was introduced in the 1930s. Retrospective studies on archived histological material found CIS lesions in women who subsequently went on to develop cervical cancer and so the precursor nature of CIS to cervical cancer came to be established. Subsequent prospective studies have confirmed these findings.[1,2]

When the Papanicolaou smear was introduced in the 1940s and abnormalities investigated, it became obvious that there were changes not amounting to CIS but still showing similar features. These lesser changes were initially referred to as 'dysplasia'. Apart from being an imprecise term covering a range of abnormalities from normal to CIS, many other terms were also in use. This resulted in confusion in management: women with CIS were usually treated by hysterectomy – sometimes radical hysterectomy – whereas those with dysplasia were often disregarded. In the 1960s, Richart introduced the term cervical intraepithelial neoplasia (CIN) and divided it into grades 1, 2 and 3. Grades 1 and 2 corresponded to mild and moderate dysplasia, respectively, and grade 3 combined severe dysplasia and CIS into one category.[3] The definition implied a continuum of change and emphasised to clinicians the concept of a single disease entity which, it was hoped, would lead to more rational management.

Table 3.1   Multistep theory of viral oncogenesis

Event	Comment
Exposure to oncogenic HPV	Common in sexually active adults
Infection with oncogenic HPV	More common in younger adults, most infections transient
Persistence of oncogenic HPV	In a minority of infected adults, infection persists, the mechanism is unknown
Immortalisation	Some cells become immortalised, accumulation of DNA damage
Transformation	Increased genetic instability results in the pre-neoplastic phenotype
Invasion	Disease is no longer confined to the epithelium

HPV = human papillomavirus

The concept of a continuum of change from CIN1 to cervical cancer has since been challenged. The process seems to be a series of discrete events starting off with human papillomavirus (HPV) infection (Table 3.1). Progression or regression depends on several factors. For practical purposes a two-stage grading is now used, with CIN1 becoming low-grade CIN, where there is a significant chance for regression, and CIN2 and CIN3 being grouped together as high-grade CIN. In North America and some European countries, this grouping has been formalised as the Bethesda classification, consisting of low-grade squamous intraepithelial lesions (LoSIL) and high-grade squamous intraepithelial lesions (HiSIL), equivalent to mild and moderate/severe dyskaryosis, respectively.

Cervical precancer has a long natural history, which is one of the reasons why it is amenable to screening. If a cancer is going to develop at all, it will take several years to do so, even from a CIN3 lesion. It is unclear why some CIN3 lesions become invasive while others stay as intraepithelial disease and it is not known how many CIN3 lesions will become invasive, since prospective studies are unethical. However, the best prospective data suggest that 30–50% of women with CIN3 would develop invasive cancer if left alone.[2]

At the other end of the spectrum, we know that a significant proportion of women with minor disease will regress to normal if left untreated. Up to 50% of women with minor cytological abnormalities will revert to normal if left alone.[4] On the other hand, one could look at the figures and say that women with mild dyskaryosis have a 16- to 47-fold increased incidence of invasive disease compared with the general female population.[5]

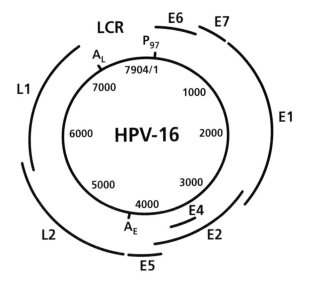

Figure 3.1 A schematic diagram of HPV

Human papillomaviruses

HPVs are small DNA viruses, about 55 nm in diameter, consisting of a single double-stranded circular chromosome of around 8000 base pairs and a 72-sided icosahedral protein coat (Figure 3.1). The chromosome is divided into early (E) and late (L) regions. The early region codes for functional proteins while the late region codes for the protein coat of the virus.

The main gene products

E6   Transforming protein that can bind to the p53 tumour suppressor
E7   Major transforming protein that binds the RB tumour suppressor
L1   Major capsid protein
L2   Minor capsid protein

Many different types of HPV have been and continue to be identified. Currently, over 100 types have been isolated. In addition to the different types there are subtypes (2–10% genomic variation compared with the prototype) and variants (less than 2% genomic variation compared with the prototype) to consider as well. Broadly speaking, they can be divided into mucosal and cutaneous types. Full virus particles are only expressed in the most superficial cells of the epithelium. As these cells are fully differentiated and cannot divide, the virus is unable to be grown in cell culture. DNA hybridisation techniques such as polymerase chain reaction (PCR) or hybrid capture detects the presence of HPV.

Genital HPVs are divided into higher-risk types (HPV-16, -18, -31, -33, -35, -45, -56, etc.) and lower risk types (HPV-6, -11, etc.) depending on their association with malignancy. Indeed, the World Health Organization has formally classified HPV-16 and -18 as carcinogenic. Regardless of the oncogenic potential, HPV should be regarded as an extremely common infection that rarely causes cancer. So how common is it? The figures vary depending on what test is used, with the highest figures being quoted where the testing has been by polymerase chain reaction (PCR). It has been estimated that 1% of American sexually active adults have visible genital warts and that 15–20% have subclinical infection detected by PCR.[6] The proportion rises to 30–40% if only young adults are considered.

Some studies even found the prevalence to be greater than 80% but these were probably flawed owing to contamination in early PCR work.[7] The figures quoted rely on testing for HPV DNA and so may not reliably assess previous infection. This can be done using serological tests seeking antibodies to capsid protein and it is likely that up to 75% of the population have been infected at some time in their lives with one or more genital HPV types.[8] These figures for prevalence of HPV and past exposure are vastly in excess of the number of cases of CIN, let alone cancer. So most infections, even with high-risk types, are transient and will be cleared in time by the host's immune responses. We know that the major immune response to HPV infection is cell mediated because women with impaired response, such as transplant patients on immunosuppression or women with HIV infection, have an increased incidence of CIN. Only the HIV patients have been found to have an increased incidence of cervical cancer, hence there must be more factors involved in carcinogenesis.[9] In contrast, women with impaired humoral immunity do not have an increased risk of HPV-associated problems.

DISEASE PREVENTION

Most, if not all, would now agree to the central role played by oncogenic HPVs in the development of CIN and cervical cancer. Furthermore, there is also some understanding of the role played by the host's immune system in preventing and eradicating infection. It was therefore inevitable that attempts would be made to exploit the virus's immunogenicity and develop vaccines to prevent infection.

There are now two commercially available vaccines, one a quadravalent vaccine directed against HPV-6, -11, -16 and -18; the second is a bivalent vaccine directed against HPV-16 and -18. The design of both vaccines exploits the ability of viral capsid proteins to self assemble into virus-like particles. The virus-like particles present the same antigenic signature to the host's immune system as a 'real' virus but as they do not contain any internal DNA they are biologically non-infective and non-transforming.

Several large randomised studies have now been completed and published and they have shown that both types of vaccine effectively increase specific immunoglobulin G, reduce or eliminate infection with type specific virus and effectively eliminate preinvasive disease related to the vaccinated subtypes.[10,11] As we believe that up to 70% of cervical cancers are the result of infections caused by either HPV-16 or -18, there is an expectation that a vaccination programme, if systematically applied, will result in a significant reduction in the burden of invasive and preinvasive disease.

There are however some unanswered questions. The duration of the effect is unknown although it would appear that it is at least 4.5 years.[12] There is no guidance as yet as to when and how often booster vaccinations may be required. Although there is some evidence that vaccinating against one subtype may provide cross-resistance with other subtypes,[13] we must still accept that up to 30% of oncogenic subtypes remain potential threats to carcinogenesis and thus it is strongly recommended that, despite the introduction of a vaccination programme, women should still be enrolled into the cervical screening programme. Whether the natural spectrum of HPVs will be altered by widespread introduction of the vaccines is also unknown. There does not appear to be any evidence as yet of an increasing prevalence of non-16/18 HPV, although this effect will probably take decades to become noticeable.

The vaccines have not been shown to confer any significant benefit to those who have already been exposed to HPV and the current focus is schoolgirls aged 12–13 years, with retrograde catch-up of older groups. Thus, by 2015, all girls between the ages of 12 and 17 years will have been offered the vaccine.

Prevention of HPV infection is a desirable goal and now, for the first time, there is clear evidence that at least some cervical cancer can be prevented. Further developments in this field are expected, particularly in the immunological intervention of those who may already have been exposed and are at risk of developing persistent disease.

IMMORTALISATION AND TRANSFORMATION

Most cells have a limited replication lifespan and can divide about 50–60 times. Infection with HPV prolongs this lifespan but eventually most of the cells stop proliferating and differentiate. Certain cell lines that have acquired genetic modifications escape differentiation and carry on dividing. This is called immortalisation. The E6 and E7 oncoproteins are necessary for this but vary in their ability to do so according to HPV type;

E6 binds to the p53 cellular protein and E7 to the RB cellular protein, both of which are cell cycle regulators.[14,15] Interfering with the cell cycle allows DNA damage to accumulate, which may result in genetic instability and transformation of the cell into a malignant cell line. This process may be accelerated by co-factors (see Chapter 1).

The NHS cervical screening programme

A nationwide organised (as opposed to opportunistic) cervical screening programme was introduced with the computerised call-and-recall system in 1988. Before this, cervical screening varied in different areas of the country. There is now a national coordinating network to ensure the adoption of common standards and working practices. In addition, a rigorous quality assurance programme insures that acceptable standards of practice prevail in cytology and in colposcopy.

Following guidance issued by the National Health Service Cervical Screening Programme (NHSCSP) in 2004,[16] strategic health authorities in England are required to offer screening to women aged 25–49 years on a 3-yearly basis and from 50 to 65 years on a 5-yearly basis. Although the time of starting screening has been controversial, the age of 25 years is consistent with World Health Organization guidance and avoids the high rates of false positives seen in teenagers and young adults as a result of transient HPV infection. The frequency and commencement point are important but perhaps less so than coverage. The effectiveness of the programme can also be judged by coverage. This is the percentage of women in the target age group (25–64 years) who have been screened in the last 5 years. If overall coverage of 80% can be achieved, the evidence suggests that a reduction in death rates of around 95% is possible in the long term. In 2007/08, the coverage of eligible women was 78.6%.[17]

Over 3.7 million smears are assessed annually in England to detect preinvasive changes. The programme has been highly effective, with 2321 new cases of cervical cancer in 2006; in 2007, there were 756 deaths attributed to cervical cancer. It has been estimated that cervical screening prevents approximately 3900 cases of cervical cancer each year.[18]

Owing to the extremely low incidence of invasive cervical cancer in women below the age of 25 years, the possible negative impact of treatment following a false positive test and because of the high prevalence of HPV infection at this age, screening of women under the age of 25 years is not justified. Of course, some women under 25 years of age are screened but this screening is opportunistic and not part of the national programme. If teenagers were screened as well, there would be a large increase in women with minor smear abnormalities requiring follow-up or investigation, the vast majority of whom would have transient HPV infection. Similarly, at the other end of the spectrum, provided that a

Table 3.2   Breakdown of cervical smear abnormalities (NHSCSP 2007/08)

Type	Incidence (%)
Borderline nuclear abnormalities	3.3
Mild dyskaryosis	1.7
Moderate dyskaryosis	0.5
Severe dyskaryosis	0.5
? Invasion or glandular abnormalities	< 0.1

woman has been adequately screened, there is no justification for continuing with screening after the age of 65 years if the smear history is normal. Indeed, some authors have questioned the validity of screening such women beyond the age of 50 years.[19,20]

Cervical cytology is not a perfect test: data from the USA have estimated the specificity to be 98% and the sensitivity only 51%.[21]

RATES OF ABNORMALITY

Before the nationwide introduction of liquid based cytology, about 92% of the smears taken were considered adequate for screening purposes. The inadequate or unsatisfactory rate has now fallen to approximately 4.7% and it was this anticipated improvement in performance that underpinned the introduction of liquid based systems. About 6% of adequate smears are 'not normal'. Most smear abnormalities are at the minor end of the spectrum (Table 3.2).

In general, the proportion of normal smears increases in older women but so does the proportion of abnormalities representing invasive cancer. Borderline changes and mild dyskaryosis are common in young women; the proportion of moderate dyskaryosis is highest for women aged 20–29 years and the proportion of severe dyskaryosis is highest in women aged 25–34 years.[22]

FURTHER INVESTIGATIONS

Women are referred for further investigation after one moderate or severe dyskaryosis smear result. Following a mild result, there is an option to repeat the smear after an interval of 6 months or refer for a colposcopic assessment. If a woman has a borderline smear it is repeated 6–12 months later and referral made on the basis of a persisting abnormality. This latter point presupposes that the cervix appears normal and that the woman has had negative smears to date. By definition, a screening test is not diagnostic but merely identifies a subgroup of the reference population at increased risk of the disease where further tests should be carried out. In this case, the reference population being screened consists of healthy asymptomatic women. As the majority of women with 'at risk' tests will either have no risk or minimal risk of developing cancer, it is vitally important to carry out the process in a way which minimises the risk of them becoming patients with disease. The screening programme has the ability to generate much psychological morbidity, which may be compounded during the course of investigation.[23]

Further investigation of smear abnormalities is by colposcopy and biopsy if indicated.

THE COLPOSCOPIC EXAMINATION

A colposcope is a low-power binocular microscope which illuminates the objective and allows for magnification from around four times to 25 times (Figure 3.2). Most devices now incorporate a green filter, which enhances visualisation of structures containing red pigment (blood vessels). In the UK it is used to assess women referred with abnormal cervical smears. In some other countries, colposcopy is considered to be a part of the routine gynaecological assessment and as such it is, in effect, a primary screen. Indeed, the colposcope was invented long before Papanicolaou and Traut

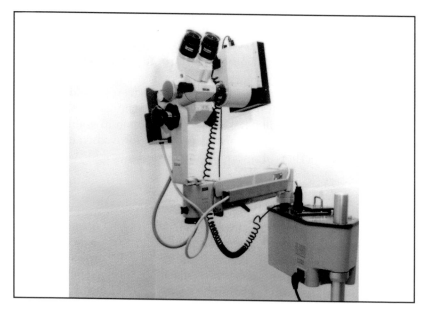

Figure 3.2 Colposcope

described cytological changes in 1943: Hans Hinselmann invented the colposcope in the 1920s in Germany as a way of detecting early invasive cancers.

Before the actual examination, time should be taken to reassure the woman, gain her confidence and listen to her questions. A brief history is taken, noting particularly the date of her last period, whether or not she smokes and what contraception she is using. The vast majority of women can be reassured prior to the examination that they are extremely unlikely to have cancer: this is very important to emphasise.

The woman is examined on a purpose-built couch in a modified lithotomy position. Her cervix is exposed with a bivalve speculum and examined with the colposcope at low magnification (×4–6). A saline-soaked cottonwool ball is then applied to the cervix, which moistens the epithelium, allowing the underlying blood vessels to be examined. Higher magnification (preferably ×16 or even ×25) is needed for this part of the examination. A green filter is a useful aid as it makes the capillaries stand out much more clearly. The various shapes of the capillaries can be studied and the intercapillary distances measured. Not all colposcopists use the saline technique but it can be particularly useful in difficult cases. Acetic acid (3% or 5%) is then applied using a cottonwool ball or by a spray. In addition to its use in diagnosis, acetic acid has a mucolytic effect and so residual mucus can be cleared away prior to the examination.

Areas of CIN will appear as varying degrees of whiteness. This is termed

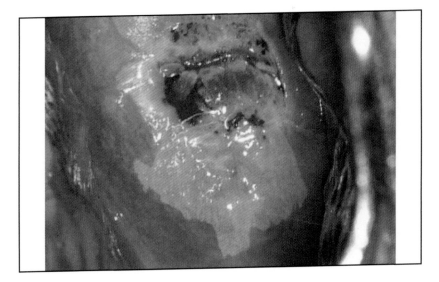

Figure 3.3 Acetowhite epithelium

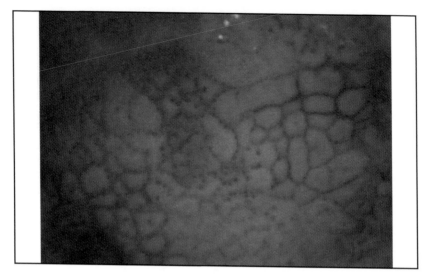

Figure 3.4 Mosaic and punctation

acetowhiteness (Figure 3.3) in contrast to areas of hyperkeratosis or leukoplakia that appear white before application of acetic acid. The exact reason why CIN tissue turns white with acetic acid is not fully understood. The cytoplasm undergoes a reversible reaction so in areas of abnormality

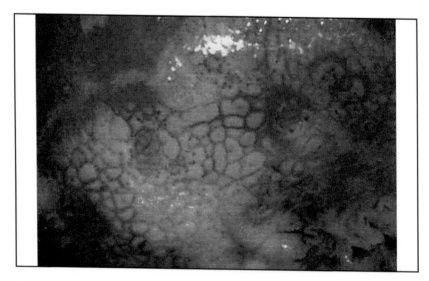

Figure 3.5 Mosaic and punctation

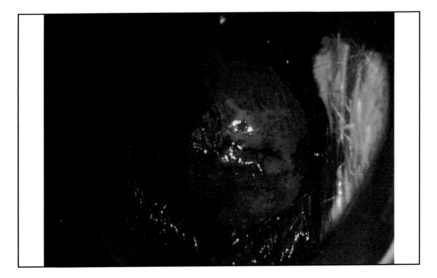

Figure 3.6 Schiller's test

where there is a high nuclear/cytoplasmic ratio in the cells the nuclei become crowded and the light from the colposcope is reflected back. Such areas will therefore appear white. However, not all areas of high nuclear density are abnormal and so not all acetowhiteness necessarily correlates with CIN: areas of regenerating epithelium, subclinical papillomavirus infection and immature metaplasia may also appear acetowhite. One of the challenges facing the colposcopist is to decide which areas of acetowhiteness truly represent premalignancy and to avoid treating benign conditions. The classical vessel patterns of CIN are punctation and mosaicism (Figures 3.4 and 3.5). Bizarrely shaped vessels suggest cancer. Another test used in the colposcopy clinic involves the application of Lugol's iodine solution to the cervix. Normal squamous epithelium contains glycogen and stains dark brown when Lugol's iodine is applied. Conversely, premalignant and malignant squamous tissue contains little or no glycogen and do not stain with iodine. This is Schiller's test: areas which are non-staining with iodine are referred to as 'Schiller positive' and those which take up iodine as 'Schiller negative' (Figure 3.6). The test is not affected by the prior application of dilute acetic acid.

The colposcopist uses many variables in forming an opinion of the underlying condition. What happens next depends on the observations made at the time and the colposcopist. There is a consensus that high-grade lesions (CIN2/3) should be treated but there is some debate about whether and when CIN1 should be treated. Some colposcopists will treat all lesions regardless of grade, whereas others will allow CIN1 lesions chance to regress. In considering which approach to adopt, the psychological impact of management policies on women should be considered. It is important that a woman is not labelled as having a sexually transmitted precancerous condition when she may only have a transient viral infection. If it is decided that treatment is needed, there are a variety of options. Broadly speaking, the abnormal tissue can be removed (excisional techniques) or it can be destroyed (ablative techniques). Removing the entire transformation zone has the advantage of allowing a large specimen to be examined: the pathologist can comment on the most severe abnormality and can assess whether all the abnormal tissue has been removed (Table 3.3). Destroying the transformation zone does not allow this, so it is mandatory to establish the diagnosis by taking a small biopsy before treatment. However, punch biopsy has been shown to be an inaccurate investigation when compared with subsequent loop excision from the same cervix.[24]

In terms of how effective the different treatment modalities are, they all achieve a 90–95% cure rate (defined by a normal smear 6 months after treatment) except cryocautery, which has a cure rate of about 85%.[25]

Table 3.3 Comparison of excisional and ablative techniques for removing abnormal tissue

Technique	Description
Excisional	
LLETZ	Removal of the transformation zone using an electrodiathermy loop (or needle). Can usually be performed under local anaesthesia
Laser cone	Removal of the transformation zone using the laser as a 'knife'. Can usually be performed under local anaesthesia
Knife cone (or cold-knife cone)	Performed under general anaesthesia
Ablative	
Electrodiathermy	Burning the transformation zone; usually performed under general anaesthesia
Cold-coagulation	A misnomer really, since the tissue is boiled by applying a probe heated to 100–120°C; performed under local anaesthesia
Cryocautery	Freezes the tissue; can be performed without anaesthesia
Laser vaporisation	Vaporises tissue; can usually be performed under local anaesthesia
Hysterectomy	The ultimate excision; may be suitable if the woman has other gynaecological problems

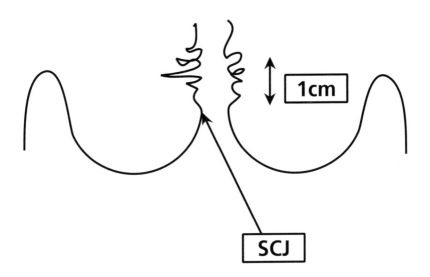

Figure 3.7 Glandular intraepithelial neoplasia; SCJ = squamocolumnar junction

Glandular premalignancy of the cervix: adenocarcinoma in situ

Glandular premalignancy of the cervix is far less common than squamous premalignancy (about 100 times less so) and is neither reliably screened for with cytology nor does it have any particular colposcopic features. The aetiological factors are the same as for squamous lesions and the two coexist in about two-thirds of cases (Figure 3.7). Compared with squamous lesions, HPV-18 is found in a higher proportion of cases.[26] Most pathologists agree that glandular precancer can be divided into low-grade and high-grade but there is more debate about whether one can distinguish three groups as in CIN (see Chapter 2). High-grade cervical glandular intraepithelial neoplasia (CGIN) is adenocarcinoma in situ (AIS). Most of these lesions arise within 1 cm of the squamocolumnar junction (Figure 3.7) but 'skip' lesions are occasionally (less than 17%) reported. Despite the latter, the condition can still be amenable to local treatment provided a large enough cone biopsy is taken (greater than 25 mm) and that the endocervical margins are free from disease. Recurrence of disease occurs in 42% of women with involved endocervical margins and 15% of women with clear margins. Follow-up of women with conservatively treated AIS must include careful endocervical cytological sampling.[27]

Vulval intraepithelial neoplasia

Premalignant changes are also recognised in other lower genital tract epithelia including the vulva. Previously, squamous vulval intraepithelial neoplasia (VIN) was categorised as VIN1, 2 and 3, according to the degree of abnormality. This bore obvious similarities to CIN. However, there was no evidence that the VIN1–3 morphologic spectrum reflected a biological continuum nor that VIN1 was a cancer precursor. The VIN2 and 3 category included two types of lesion, which differed in morphology, biology and clinical features. The first type of VIN, usual type (warty, basaloid and mixed), is HPV-related in most cases. Invasive squamous carcinomas of warty or basaloid type are associated with VIN, usual type. The second type of VIN, differentiated type, is seen particularly in older women with lichen sclerosus and/or squamous cell hyperplasia in some cases. Neither VIN, differentiated type, nor associated keratinising squamous-cell carcinoma is HPV-related. The term VIN should apply only to histologically high-grade squamous lesions (former terms, VIN2 and VIN3 and differentiated VIN3). The term VIN1 should no longer be used. Two categories should describe squamous VIN: VIN, usual type (encompassing former VIN2 and 3 of warty, basaloid and mixed types) and VIN, differentiated type (VIN3, differentiated type).[28]

VIN is not a common disease but it appears to be increasing particularly in younger women (although part of the reason for this may be more effective detection rather than a genuine increase).[29] The association with HPV infection is strong (although not as strong as for CIN), particularly in young women, and these women may have other intraepithelial neoplasias of the anogenital tract (a 'field change'). Conclusions drawn from earlier series and publications need to be interpreted with caution as few separated out the HPV from the non-HPV types of VIN. In effect, there are two distinct disease processes.

VIN mainly affects the labia minora and the perineum and can take a variety of forms, which accounts for the difficulty in diagnosis. If there are associated and obvious features of lichen sclerosus or squamous-cell hyperplasia then differentiated VIN should be considered, although usual-type VIN can also occur in these patients. The woman may complain of itching (vulval pruritus), in about 40% of cases, or soreness and burning.[30] A substantial number, however, will be asymptomatic and the abnormality will be a chance finding on examination. The lesions may be unifocal or multifocal and there may be extension to the perianal and anal mucosa (Figure 3.8).

Diagnosis is made by examining the vulva with a good light source (such as with the colposcope at low magnification). Acetic acid may be used but the changes take longer to occur than for CIN and are certainly not specific with normal vulval epithelium also staining acetowhite.[31]

Clinical suspicions are confirmed by biopsy. Management has become much more conservative in view of the relatively low invasive potential and the physical and psychological scarring that will be inflicted with extensive vulval surgery. Unfortunately, current treatments for VIN are suboptimal in

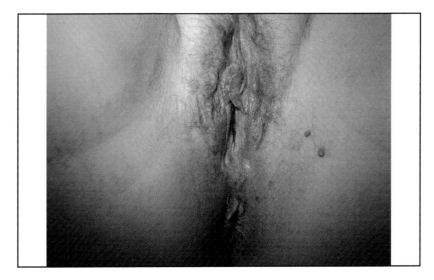

Figure 3.8 Mutifocal VIN

terms of their poor clinical response rates and high relapse rates. The high recurrence rates following many therapies may reflect the fact that they fail to remove the reservoir of HPV present in the vulval skin and/or epigenetic changes in the surrounding lichen sclerosus of differentiated VIN. Lesions can be treated by local excision or destruction using laser or diathermy. The indications to offer treatment include new or deteriorating symptoms not controlled by non-surgical means or a suspicion of invasion. Differentiated VIN is alleged to have a higher risk of progression[32] and, in the author's clinic, excision is recommended if differentiated VIN is suspected and excision in all cases where a suspicion of invasion must be excluded.

Recurrences of 39% and 70% have been described after surgical excision and laser ablation, respectively.[33,34] If a woman has VIN, the rest of the lower genital tract should be carefully examined, as there is an increased risk of intraepithelial neoplasia at other sites.

Vaginal intraepithelial neoplasia

Vaginal intraepithelial neoplasia (VAIN) is extremely uncommon (about 150 times less common than CIN). In 70% of cases of VAIN there will be associated CIN. The average age of the woman with VAIN tends to be greater than for CIN. The major predisposing factor is the same, namely oncogenic HPV, but the reason for the lower incidence is the relative stability of the epithelium compared with the metaplastic cervical epithelium. Women exposed to diethylstilbestrol in utero have a higher incidence of VAIN as, here, the areas of metaplastic transformation extend on to the vagina. Around 25% of women with VAIN will have had a hysterectomy previously, either for CIN or benign conditions. It is now recommended that if a woman has not had a negative smear within the prescribed screening interval before hysterectomy then cytology should be performed. If there is any doubt, a preoperative colposcopy can be performed first to determine if there is an atypical transformation zone and second to determine whether there is a vaginal extension. If there is evidence of an atypical transformation zone extending to the vagina then a cuff of vagina can be taken before removal of the uterine specimen, insuring that all atypical epithelium is removed with the uterine specimen.

Like CIN, VAIN is graded 1–3 but, in common with VIN, the invasive potential is less than for CIN. Treatment of VAIN3 is by surgical excision. This may necessitate a combined abdominovaginal approach to excise the vaginal vault. Chemosurgery using 5-fluorouracil before diathermy ablation is an experimental treatment that has shown some promising results. Radiotherapy is an alternative treatment for women who may not be suitable for surgery. Lower grades can be observed. For women who have had hysterectomy where VAIN is seen at the vaginal vault, there may still be disease buried above the vault in the cuff that was closed over at hysterectomy.

KEY POINTS

- CIN has a long natural history.
- HPV infection is extremely common but rarely causes cancer.
- A vaccination programme against HPV-16 and -18 may result in a significant reduction in cervical cancer incidence over time.
- Organised cervical cytology screening is effective in reducing the incidence of cervical cancer but is very expensive and may cause significant psychological morbidity.
- Screening is not justified for teenagers and women below the age of 25 years.
- Local treatment for CIN is highly effective.
- Vaginal and vulval intraepithelial neoplasias are much less common and appear to have less invasive potential than CIN.

References

1. Koss LG, Stewart FW, Foote FW, Jordan JM, Badger GM, Day E. Some histological aspects of the behaviour of epidermoid carcinoma in situ and related lesions of the uterine cervix: a long-term prospective study. *Cancer* 1963;16:1160–211.

2. McIndoe WA, McLean MR, Jones RW, Mullins PR. The invasive potential of carcinoma in situ of the cervix. *Obstet Gynecol* 1984;64:451–8.

3. Richart RM. Natural history of cervical intraepithelial neoplasia. *Clin Obstet Gynecol* 1967;10:748–84.

4. Robertson JH, Woodend BE, Crozier EH, Hutchinson J. Risk of cervical cancer associated with mild dyskaryosis. *BMJ* 1988;297:18–21.

5. Soutter WP. The management of a mildly dyskaryotic smear: immediate referral to colposcopy is safer. *BMJ* 1994;309:591–2.

6. Koutsky L Epidemiology of genital human papillomavirus infection. *Am J Med* 1997;102(5A):3–8.

7. Young LS, Bevan IS, Johnson MA, Blomfield PI, Bromidge T, Maitland NJ, *et al.* The polymerase chain reaction: a new epidemiological tool for investigating cervical human papillomavirus infection. *BMJ* 1989;298:14–18.

8. Syrjanen K, Syrjanen S. Epidemiology of human papilloma virus infections and genital neoplasia. *Scand J Infect Dis* 1990;69 Suppl:7–17.

9. Alloub MI, Barr BB, McLaren KM, Smith IW, Bunney MH, Smart GE. Human papillomavirus infection and cervical intraepithelial neoplasia in women with renal allografts. *BMJ* 1992;298:153–6.

10. Paavonen J, Jenkins D, Bosch FX, Naud P, Salmerón J, Wheeler CM, *et al.* Efficacy of a prophylactic adjuvanted bivalent L1 virus-like-particle vaccine against infection with human papillomavirus types 16 and 18 in young women: an interim analysis of a phase III double-blind, randomised controlled trial. *Lancet* 2007;369:2161–70.

11. Joura EA, Leodolter S, Hernandez-Avila M, Wheeler CM, Perez G, Koutsky LA, *et al.* Efficacy of a quadrivalent prophylactic human papillomavirus (types 6, 11, 16, and 18) L1 virus-like-particle vaccine against high-grade vulval and vaginal lesions: a combined analysis of three randomised clinical trials. *Lancet* 2007;369:1693–702.

12. Harper DM, Franco EL, Wheeler CM, Moscicki AB, Romanowski B, Roteli-Martins CM, *et al.* Sustained efficacy up to 4.5 years of a bivalent L1 virus-like particle vaccine against human papillomavirus types 16 and 18: follow-up from a randomised control trial. *Lancet* 2006;367:1247–55.

13. Jenkins D. A review of cross-protection against oncogenic HPV by an HPV-16/18 AS04-adjuvanted cervical cancer vaccine: importance of virological and clinical endpoints and implications for mass vaccination in cervical cancer prevention. *Gynecol Oncol* 2008;110(3 Suppl 1):S18–25.

14. Werness BA, Levine AJ, Howley PM. Association of human papillomavirus types 16 and 18 E6 proteins with p53. *Science* 1990;248:76–9.

15. White E. p53 guardian of Rb. *Nature* 1994;371:21–2.

16. National Health Service Cancer Screening Programmes. *Colposcopy and Programme Management: Guidelines for the NHS Cervical Screening Programme.* NHSCSP Publication No. 20. Sheffield: NHSCSP; 2004 [www.cancerscreening.nhs.uk/cervical/publications/nhscsp20.html].

17. National Health Service Information Centre. *Cervical Screening Programme, England 2007–08.* London: Health and Social Care Information Centre; 2008 [www.ic.nhs.uk/statistics-and-data-collections/screening/cervical-cancer/cervical-screening-programme-2007-08-%5Bns%5D].

18. Peto J, Gilham C, Fletcher O, Matthews FE., The cervical cancer epidemic that screening has prevented in the UK. *Lancet* 2004;364:249–56.

19. Hakama M, Miller AB, Day NE, editors. *Screening for Cancer of the Uterine Cervix.* Lyon: International Agency for Research on Cancer; 1986.

20. Van Wijngaarden WJ, Duncan ID. Rationale for stopping cervical screening in women over 50. *BMJ* 1993;306:967–7.

21. Agency for Health Care Research and Quality. Evaluation of Cervical Cytology: Evidence Report. Technology Assessment No. 5, January 1999 [www.ahrq. gov/clinic/epcsums/cervsumm.htm].

22. Department of Health. *Cervical Screening Programme, England:2000–01.* Statistical Bulletin 2001/22. London: DH; 2001 [www.dh.gov.uk/en/ Publicationsandstatistics/Publications/PublicationsStatistics/DH_4006068].

23. Marteau TM, Walker PB, Giles J, Smail M. Anxieties in women undergoing colposcopy. *Br J Obstet Gynaecol* 1990;97:859–61.

24. Buxton EJ, Luesley DM, Shafi MI, Rollason T. Colposcopically directed punch biopsy: a potentially misleading investigation. *Br J Obstet Gynaecol* 1991;98:1273–6.

25. Martin-Hirsch PL, Paraskevaidis E, Kitchener H. Surgery for cervical intraepithelial neoplasia. *Cochrane Database Syst Rev* 2001;(4).

26. Bekkers RL, Bulten J, Wiersma-van Tilburg A, Mravunac M, Schijf CP, *et al.* Coexisting high-grade glandular and squamous cervical lesions and human papillomavirus infections. *Br J Cancer* 2003;89:886–90.

27. Etherington IJ, Luesley DM. Adenocarcinoma in situ of the cervix: controversies in diagnosis and treatment. *J Low Genit Tract Dis* 2001;5:94–8.

28. Sideri M, Jones RW, Wilkinson EJ, Preti M, Heller DS, Scurry J, *et al.* Squamous vulvar intraepithelial neoplasia: 2004 modified terminology, ISSVD Vulvar Oncology Subcommittee. *J Reprod Med* 2005;50:807–10.

29. Jones RW, Baranyai J, Stables S. Trends in squamous cell carcinoma of the vulva: the influence of vulvar intraepithelial neoplasia. *Obstet Gynecol* 1997;90:448–52.

30. Campion MJ, Singer A. Vulvar intraepithelial neoplasia: clinical review. *Genitourin Med* 1987;63:147–52.

31. van Beurden M, van der Vange N, de Craen AJ, Tjong-A-Hung SP, ten Kate FJ, ter Schegget J, *et al.* Normal findings in vulvar examination and vulvoscopy. *Br J Obstet Gynaecol* 1997;104:320–4.

32. Eva LJ, Ganesan R, Chan KK, Honest H, Luesley DM. Differentiated-type vulval intraepithelial neoplasia has a high-risk association with vulval squamous cell carcinoma. *Int J Gynecol Cancer* 2009;19:741–4.

33. DiSaia PJ, Rich WM. Surgical approach to multifocal carcinoma in situ of the vulva. *Am J Obstet Gynecol* 1981;140:136–45.

34. Townsend DE, Levine RU, Richart RM, Crum CP, Petrilli ES. Management of vulvar intraepithelial neoplasia by carbon dioxide laser. *Obstet Gynecol* 1982;60:49–52.

4 Radiological assessment

Introduction

Radiological assessment forms an integral part of the multidisciplinary management of gynaecological cancers. This chapter describes the role of imaging modalities in gynaecological cancer.

Ovarian cancer

There are two main goals of imaging in this area:[1]

- to differentiate benign from malignant ovarian masses
- to aid management in patients with ovarian malignancy.

DIFFERENTIATING BENIGN FROM MALIGNANT OVARIAN MASSES

Pelvic ultrasound is the primary imaging modality in the assessment of ovarian masses. The transvaginal route is preferred to the transabdominal, as the higher-frequency probes used have better resolution, giving a more detailed assessment of the mass. High-frequency probes have a limited range: a maximum depth of view 6–10 cm, so the two techniques are used in conjunction. This is particularly important if the mass is large.

There are ultrasonic features which correlate with malignancy and these have been incorporated into the risk of malignancy index (RMI). The RMI is used to predict whether an ovarian mass is malignant. As discussed in Chapter 9, the RMI is based on the findings at ultrasound, the pre- or post-menopausal state and the serum CA125 level.

The most significant pointer of malignancy at ultrasound is an indication of solid elements, particularly if blood flow can be demonstrated within the ovary by using colour or power Doppler. Blood clot and collections can also simulate solid masses but will have no blood flow. Waveform analysis (resistive index and pulsatility index) was previously used to differentiate benign from malignant masses but subsequent studies brought this into question and it no longer forms part of the assessment.[2]

Ultrasound scans are scored one point for each of the following characteristics:

- multilocular cyst
- solid areas within the mass
- bilateral lesions
- ascites
- evidence of intra-abdominal metastasis (Figures 4.1 and 4.2).

Patients with an RMI greater than 200 should be referred to a gynaecological cancer centre. The RMI has weaknesses and should not be used when there is clear evidence of tumour spread at ultrasound. Unilocular simple cystic masses of less than 5 cm are likely to be benign and in the context of a normal serum CA125 measurement they can be managed conservatively.[3]

Magnetic resonance imaging (MRI) is playing an increasingly important role in the evaluation of the indeterminate ovarian mass seen at ultrasound. Ultrasound and MRI are both sensitive but MRI is more specific, as ultrasound has a higher false positive rate.[4] MRI can readily characterise haemorrhagic cysts, endometriomas, dermoids, ovarian fibromas and pedunculated fibroids, all of which can give false positive features of tumour at ultrasound. MRI is most valuable when the serum

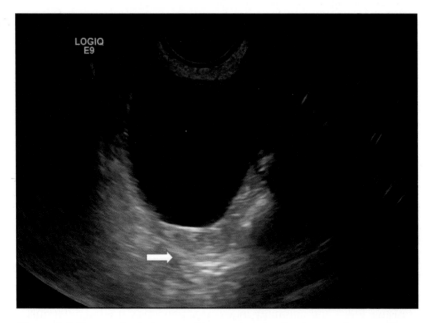

Figure 4.1 Transvaginal ultrasound image showing benign ovarian cyst. Note the following features which suggest a simple cyst: round or oval shape, well-defined smooth wall, anechoic and increased through transmission posterior to the cyst (arrow)

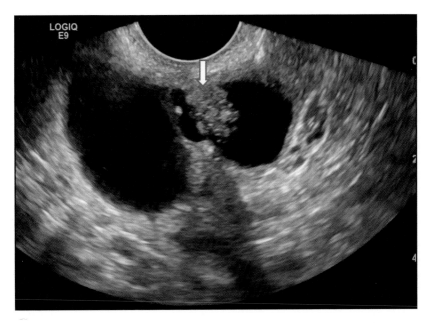

Figure 4.2 Transvaginal ultrasound image showing ovarian cyst with features suspicious of malignancy; there is a solid papillary projection (arrow) and thick septa

CA125 level is normal or only slightly elevated. The use of MRI in this context can reduce the number of women undergoing cancer surgery in specialist units; rather, they can be managed in the local cancer unit by a general gynaecologist.[5]

PATIENTS WITH FEATURES IN KEEPING WITH MALIGNANCY AT ULTRASOUND

In women with ultrasonic evidence of malignancy, either within the ovary or where there is ascites, generally indicating peritoneal spread of tumour, further assessment with contrast-enhanced computed tomography (CT) of the abdomen and pelvis should be performed. Metastatic disease to the chest is frequently a late feature, usually manifesting as pleural effusions secondary to pleural metastasis. CT of the chest at initial staging is not always performed. Some centres do this only if pleural effusions are demonstrated by chest X-ray or on abdominal CT (which includes the costophrenic areas), while others include it so that there is a baseline available and argue it is useful as, in up to 10% of cases, the final diagnosis will be something other than ovarian cancer.

The main questions for CT to answer in a woman with suspected ovarian cancer is whether the tumour can be successfully debulked at primary surgery or whether a course of neoadjuvant chemotherapy prior to cytoreductive surgery is warranted. Features on CT which are likely to render the patient inoperable include:

- serosal spread around the liver and spleen
- visceral metastasis
- deposits in the root of the small bowel mesentery
- retroperitoneal lymphadenopathy, particularly above the level of the renal vessels
- bulky peritoneal deposits greater than 2 cm in diameter
- extensive bowel involvement (Figure 4.3a,b).[6]

It is important to identify ureteric and bowel involvement preoperatively, as the expertise of a urologist or colorectal surgeon may be required. The other important role of imaging is to considerer whether the ovarian masses may represent metastatic spread from primary tumours such as breast, colon, pancreas and stomach.

When CT demonstrates that primary surgery is inappropriate,

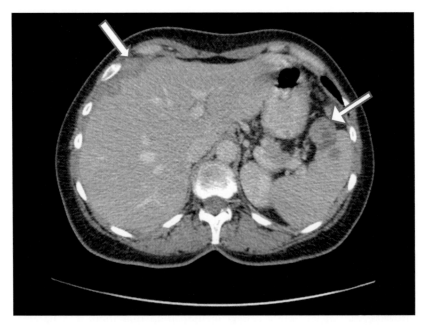

Figure 4.3a Axial CT image showing inoperable ovarian cancer; peritoneal tumour deposits are demonstrated around the liver and spleen (arrows)

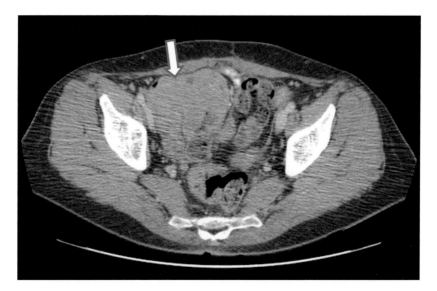

Figure 4.3b Axial CT image showing inoperable ovarian cancer; there is a large volume tumour on the right side of the pelvis (arrow) which is intimately related to bowel

histological confirmation of the diagnosis is mandatory before chemotherapy to ensure that the correct chemotherapy regimen is used. As highlighted previously, peritoneal spread from other tumours can mimic ovarian cancer. Image-guided biopsy is the mainstay of gaining a tissue sample. Ultrasound or CT-guided biopsies of peritoneal deposits can be performed and the transvaginal ultrasound approach can also be used for isolated pelvic disease.

MONITORING THERAPY AND RECURRENT DISEASE

CT of the abdomen and pelvis is the workhorse for monitoring disease response to chemotherapy and is based on the Response Evaluation Criteria In Solid Tumors (RECIST) rules. The role of chest CT in this setting is again questionable. Supradiaphragmatic disease in the absence of abdominopelvic disease is rare and should therefore only be performed if there is evidence of pleural effusions.

There is no place for routine imaging in the follow-up of treated ovarian cancer; that is, following a complete treatment response or patients who are in remission. CT, however, is indicated in the assessment of progressive disease or suspicion of disease relapse. If CT is negative following an elevated serum CA125 with clinical suspicion of relapse, there are a number of options which include watch-and-wait and interval scans.

Positron emission tomography (PET) has been shown to be of value in this context.[7]

COMPLICATIONS

Common complications of advanced ovarian cancer include large volume ascites, bowel obstruction and urinary problems secondary to either compression effects on the bladder or, less commonly, ureteric obstruction. CT is the best modality for diagnosing these problems. In the context of bowel obstruction, CT can help identify the small group of patients who would benefit from surgery, where a localised tumour mass causes obstruction rather than the more common finding of diffuse bowel involvement.

Symptomatic ascites should be managed with drainage after a suitable site has been marked with ultrasound. In the palliative setting when patients require frequent drainage (every 2–3 weeks or less) then insertion of a long-term ascitic drain should be considered. These drains are inserted under ultrasound guidance by a radiologist and tunnelled under the skin to reduce the risk of infection. They can be left in for as long as they remain patent. Patients should be counselled to make sure they are happy with the idea of a permanent drain.

Cervical cancer

Imaging has a vital role to play in determining correct management of cervical cancer, at initial staging, recurrent disease and looking for complications. The FIGO staging of cervical cancer is based on clinical examination. Lymph node spread and the findings at MRI and CT do not alter this.

Patients with cervical cancer have two main treatment options: surgery or primary chemoradiotherapy. The two main factors which determine choice of treatment are parametrial extension and lymph node involvement. The role of imaging is to address these two issues.

WHO SHOULD HAVE IMAGING?

Patients with macroscopically visible cancer clinically confined to the cervix should have a pelvic MRI. Patients with stage IB1 tumours and above should have a CT of the chest and abdomen to exclude distant spread of disease. Imaging can help to answer the following questions, some of which will determine whether the patient is suitable for an operation:

- tumour volume
- parametrical extension
- confirming that the tumour is confined to the cervix
- nodal status.

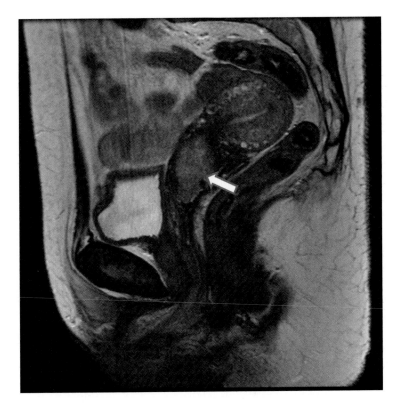

Figure 4.4 Sagittal T2 weighted image demonstrating a cervical cancer. The uterus is retroverted. The cervical canal is expanded by intermediate signal intensity tumour (arrow)

TUMOUR VOLUME

Tumour volume is assessed at MRI. Cervical tumour is a high signal on T2-weighted images compared with the normal low signal cervical stroma (Figure 4.4). When the tumour is small, it can be difficult to distinguish tumour from post-biopsy changes and, where possible, there should be a 10-day interval before MRI. The maximal tumour dimension is taken. Four centimetres is the normal cut off for operability.

Tumour confined to the cervix

Trachelectomy (uterine preservation treatment) may be considered for stage IA or IB tumours in women who wish to conserve fertility. MRI is performed preoperatively to assess tumour size and location. Exclusion criteria include tumours greater than 2 cm in size and involvement of the uterine isthmus,[8] both of which can be accurately assessed at MRI.

Parametrial extension

Parametrial involvement is determined by assessment of the cervical stromal ring. Thin sections are performed through the cervix perpendicular to the long axis of the cervix. Normal cervical stroma is seen as an intact low signal ring. This appearance on MRI has a high negative predictive value for parametrial invasion (Figure 4.4). When parametrial extension is present, the low signal ring is disrupted and there is an irregular infiltrating margin between tumour and the parametrium. One of the pitfalls of MRI, however, is that early parametrial extension is difficult to identify and complete loss of the low signal cervical ring does not always indicate definite parametrial extension.

CONFIRMING THAT THE TUMOUR IS CONFINED TO THE CERVIX

MRI can accurately assess invasion into local structures, such as the vagina, bladder and rectum, and extension to the pelvic side wall. Uterine extension is also important to document, as this is a poor prognostic indicator and commonly associated with nodal spread.[9]

A normal appearance of the bladder and rectum on MRI examination obviates the need for cystoscopy or sigmoidoscopy. If there is suspicion of involvement at imaging then cystoscopy or sigmoidoscopy with a view to biopsy should be performed. Intravenous urograms are no longer performed, as CT and MRI provide accurate assessment of ureteric involvement and hydronephrosis while giving additional information not gained at urography.

NODAL STATUS

As discussed, nodal status does not form part of the FIGO classification. Accurate assessment of lymph node status is vital, though, for two reasons:

1. Involved nodes generally would render the patient inoperable. When tumour has spread to lymph nodes, primary chemotherapy is preferred to hysterectomy followed by chemotherapy, as this so called 'trimodality therapy' incurs greater morbidity with no improvement in outcome.[10]
2. It is the single biggest predictor of long term survival.

A 1-cm cut-off point is used before a node is deemed to be pathological. MRI and CT have high specificity (94%) but low sensitivity of approximately 40–60%, as they fail to pick up deposits in normal sized nodes.[11] CT and MRI have replaced lymphangiography, which is more invasive and less sensitive.

PET is a newer modality and is more accurate than CT and MRI at assessing nodal status. It is more sensitive (75%) and specific (100%) than MRI. It is currently finding its place in the imaging algorithm. The Scottish

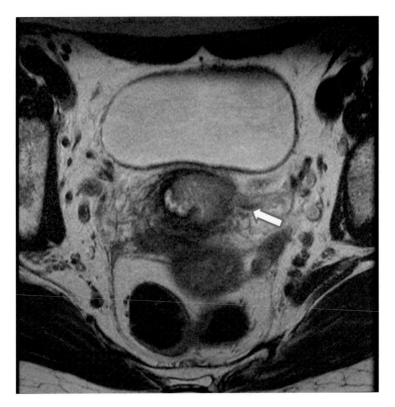

Figure 4.5 Transaxial T2 WI image demonstrating cervical tumour. The low signal cervical stroma is breached on the left side and tumour extends into the parametrium (arrow)

Intercollegiate Guidelines Network guidelines recommend its use in patients not suitable for surgery in whom radical chemoradiotherapy is being considered, as this group of women is statistically more likely to have nodal involvement or metastatic disease than those women who are fit for surgery (Figure 4.5).[12]

For patients with advanced disease clinically (that is, FIGO stage IV) CT of the chest, abdomen and pelvis is recommended and MRI is not routinely indicated.

RADIOTHERAPY

CT is the standard imaging method for radiotherapy planning but has inferior soft tissue contrast when compared with MRI. MRI is used to monitor response to radiotherapy looking for a reduction in tumour volume and reduction and resolution of any previously enlarged pelvic lymph nodes. PET has also been shown to be accurate in monitoring therapy response.[7]

RECURRENT DISEASE AND COMPLICATIONS

Approximately one-third of patients with invasive cervical cancer will develop recurrent disease. Recurrence is frequently central – involving the vaginal vault post-surgery and uterus post-chemoradiotherapy. Recurrence may also occur at the pelvic side wall and distant sites of spread include liver and lung metastasis. MRI and CT are equally good at demonstrating local recurrence. MRI is better at differentiating radiation fibrosis and postoperative scar tissue from recurrent tumour but this can still remain a difficult assessment. MRI also provides more detailed assessment of pelvic soft tissue structures, which enables accurate surgical planning. PET has a higher sensitivity for detecting recurrent tumour than CT or MRI and is likely to play an increasing role in this area.[13] PET should be performed before pelvic exenteration, as it frequently detects unsuspected distant metastatic disease which renders curative surgery fruitless (Figure 4.6).[12] Complications of radiotherapy, such as rectovaginal and vesicovaginal fistula, are best demonstrated with MRI.

Endometrial cancer

Transvaginal ultrasound is the initial investigation in a woman with post-menopausal bleeding. Endometrial thickness is assessed and the threshold for intervention is 5 mm. Ultrasound has a 96% sensitivity for detection of endometrial cancer[14] and a high negative predictive value for excluding endometrial cancer. If the endometrial thickness is 5 mm or greater, endometrial sampling is required, as ultrasound cannot reliably differentiate cancer from benign aetiologies such as polyps and hyperplasia (Figure 4.7).

The role of cross-sectional imaging in the management of endometrial cancer has changed as a result of the ASTEC trial (A Study in the Treatment of Endometrial Cancer).[15] Previously, many women underwent MRI to assess the depth of myometrial invasion, as this correlates with the likelihood of lymph node metastasis and the need for lymphadenectomy. However, the ASTEC trial concluded that lymph node spread is more closely linked to tumour grade.[15] Tumour grade and cell type have now become the determining factors in selecting patients for lymphadenectomy. Patients with grade I and II tumours generally need no further imaging before surgery. Patients with high-grade tumours (grade III) or aggressive cell types such as clear-cell, serous and undifferentiated tumours, are staged with CT of the chest, abdomen and pelvis to look for evidence of distant spread.

Cervical involvement is important to determine preoperatively, as this will affect surgical procedure (simple hysterectomy or Wertheim's).

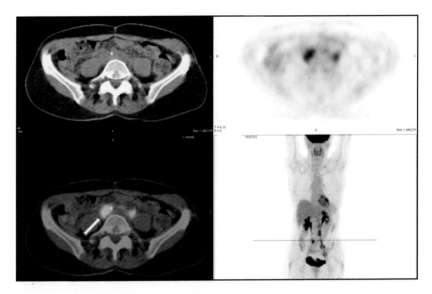

Figure 4.6 PET, CT and fused data sets are shown; there are enlarged FDG avid right-sided low para-aortic lymph nodes (arrow); the uptake at the same level on the left is in the ureter

Although some assessment of the cervix can be made with ultrasound, MRI is more sensitive and should be requested in patients where this is suspected either clinically or at ultrasound.

As CT has poor soft tissue contrast and cannot accurately assess the endometrium, its role is in detecting spread beyond the uterus, detecting both nodal and distant spread.

MRI is invaluable in radiotherapy planning, allowing tumour volumes to be more accurately assessed than at CT. It influences the choice of radiotherapy, brachytherapy (uterine confined) or external beam therapy.

MRI and CT both have a role to play in the assessment of recurrent disease. MRI is advocated for assessment of locally recurrent disease in the pelvis before surgery and CT for the assessment of possible distant spread. Local recurrence may present as a pelvic mass in the hysterectomy bed or as pelvic or retroperitoneal lymphadenopathy. Fluorodeoxyglucose (18F) has also been assessed in a small series of patients, with promising results.[16]

Rarer gynaecological tumours

SARCOMAS

Mixed müllerian tumours account for 5% of uterine tumours. Local spread is best assessed at MRI and CT performed to look for distant spread. They can be indistinguishable from endometrial carcinomas on imaging.

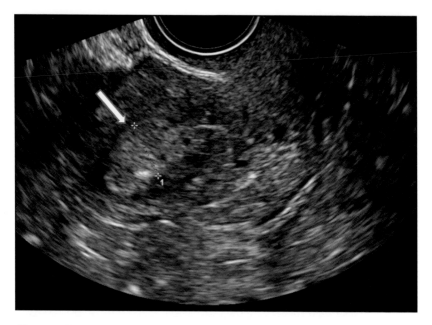

Figure 4.7 Transvaginal ultrasound image of the uterus in sagittal section; the endometrium is thickened and heterogeneous (arrow) measuring 11 mm

Leiomyosarcomas account for 1% of all uterine tumours. They usually arise de novo rather than by malignant transformation of a fibroid. It is not possible to accurately distinguish a degenerating fibroid from a leiomyosarcoma on any imaging modality and the diagnosis is a histological one but sarcoma should be considered when the mass has an irregular outline and heterogeneous signal. Detecting metastatic spread to bone, lung and lymph nodes is performed with CT.

GESTATIONAL TROPHOBLASTIC TUMOUR

The main role of imaging is to confirm the presence of a mixed echogenic mass with cystic vascular channels within the uterus. The modality of choice is Doppler ultrasound as it is an easy and non-invasive technique. In addition, the marked hypervascularity of these lesions make it very sensitive with power Doppler. Ultrasound will also exclude a viable pregnancy. The majority of uncomplicated cases of gestational trophoblastic tumour (GTT) have no further imaging except a chest X-ray. CT and MRI are performed in cases which are chemoresistant or have a high FIGO score. All cases of GTT should be referred to a national referral centre.

VAGINAL CANCER

Imaging is not needed in what are thought to be early stage I tumours clinically. MRI is helpful with stage II and III tumours and is preferred to CT, in view of its better soft tissue contrast. It is used to help surgical treatment planning and to look for adenopathy. CT is performed in stage IV disease and also has a role in radiotherapy planning in more advanced stages of disease.

VULVAL CANCER

Cancer of the vulva accounts for about 3–5% of primary gynaecological malignancies. The single most important prognostic factor is the presence or absence of nodal metastases. Preoperative assessment of the primary tumour is best performed with a MRI, which allows evaluation of the tumour's deeper extent and its relation to the adjacent pelvic structures such as the anal sphincters. MRI also provides good assessment of the inguinal and pelvic lymph nodes, although the assessment of more distal lymphadenopathy is better with a CT scan. More increasingly, PET is finding a role, particularly in helping to determine suitability for more extensive lymph node dissection and radiotherapy.

References

1. Spencer J, Forstner R, Hricak H. Investigating women with suspected ovarian cancer. *Gynecol Oncol* 2008;108:262–4.
2. Royal College of Obstetricians and Gynaecologists. *Ovarian Cysts in Postmenopausal Women*. Green-top Guideline No. 34. London: RCOG; 2003 [www.rcog.org.uk/womens-health/clinical-guidance/ovarian-cysts-postmenopausal-women-green-top-34].
3. Roman LD, Muderspach LI, Stein SM, Laifer-Narin S, Groshen S, Morrow CP. Pelvic examination, tumour marker level, and grey-scale and Doppler sonography in the prediction of pelvic cancer. *Obstet Gynecol* 1997;89:493–500.
4. Sohaib SA, Mills TD, Sahdev A, Webb JA, Vantrappen PO, Jacobs IJ, *et al*. The role of magnetic resonance imaging and ultrasound in women with adnexal masses. *Clin Radiol* 2005;60:340–8.
5. Spencer J. Magnetic resonance (MR) imaging of suspected ovarian cancer. *BJOG* 2008;115:811–13.
6. Meyer J, Kennedy A, Friedmen R. Ovarian carcinoma: value of CT in predicting success of debulking surgery. *Am J Radiol* 1995;165:875–8.
7. Schwarz JK, Grigsby PW, Dehdashti F, Delbeke D. The role of FDG PET in assessing therapy response in cancer of the cervix and ovaries. *J Nucl Med* 2009; 50(5 Suppl):65s–73s.
8. Morice P, Petrow P, Pomel C. Radical trachelectomy: a need for a careful preoperative assessment. *Am J Obstet Gynecol* 2003;189:1515.

9. Hope A, Saha P, Grigsby P. FDG-PET in carcinoma of the uterine cervix with endometrial extension. *Cancer* 2006:106:196–200.

10 Landoni F, Maneo A, Colombo A, Placa F, Milani R, Perego P, *et al*. Randomised study of radical surgery versus radiotherapy for stage 1b–IIA cervical cancer. *Lancet* 1997;350:535–40.

11. Hricak H, Gatsonis C, Coakley FV, Snyder B, Reinhold C, Schwartz LH, *et al*. Early invasive cervical cancer: CT and MR imaging in preoperative evaluation. ACRIN/GOG comparative study of diagnostic performance and interobserver variability. *Radiology* 2007;245:491–8.

12. Scottish Intercollegiate Guidelines Network. *Management of Cervical Cancer*. A national clinical guideline, No. 99. Edinburgh: SIGN; 2008 [www.sign.ac.uk/guidelines/fulltext/99/index.html].

13. Havrilesky LJ, Wong TZ, Secord AA, Berchuck A, Clarke-Pearson DL, Jones EL. The role of PET scanning in the detection of recurrent cervical cancer. *Gynecol Oncol* 2003;90:186–90.

14. Smith-Bindman R, Kerlikowske K, Feldstein VA, Subak L, Scheidler J, Segal M, *et al*. Endovaginal ultrasound to exclude endometrial cancer and other endometrial abnormalities. *JAMA* 1998;280:1510–17.

15. ASTEC/EN.5 Study Group, Blake P, Swart AM, Orton J, Kitchener H, Whelan T, Lukka H, *et al*. Adjuvant external beam radiotherapy in the treatment of endometrial cancer (MRC ASTEC and NCIC CTG EN.5 randomised trials): pooled trial results, systematic review, and meta-analysis. *Lancet* 2009;373:137–46.

16. Saga T, Higashi T, Ishimori T, Mamede M, Nakamoto Y, Mukai T, *et al*. Clinical value of FDG-PET in the follow up of post-operative patients with endometrial cancer. *Ann Nucl Med* 2003;17:197–203.

5 Surgical principles

Introduction

Surgery has various applications in the management of cancer. These roles may change according to the site and extent of the tumour, the general health of the individual and the patient's wishes. In general, the roles that can be performed by surgery include:

- diagnosis
- staging
- treatment
- reconstruction
- palliation.

Diagnosis

In general, the diagnosis of a cancer will be made by means of a biopsy taken either as an outpatient procedure or under general anaesthesia, such as hysteroscopy, cervical biopsy or vulval biopsy. This investigation may also incorporate part of the staging procedure. For ovarian cancer, the definitive diagnosis may be confirmed only at laparotomy or when the histology results from laparotomy are available. Sometimes the diagnosis is made by means of interventional radiology, such as core biopsy of a distant metastasis.

Staging

Staging is a process whereby the extent of the disease at presentation is defined using agreed international guidelines. Most gynaecologists use the FIGO staging system (Appendix 1) but the TNM system (tumour, nodes, metastases) is also used, particularly with vulval cancer (see Chapter 12). Staging may be clinical or surgical. Clinical staging includes:

- examination under anaesthesia
- tumour biopsy
- cystoscopy (± biopsy)
- sigmoidoscopy (± biopsy)

- endometrial curettage
- chest X-ray
- intravenous urogram
- skeletal X-ray.

Cervical cancer is clinically staged (see Chapter 11) because a significant number of patients will not undergo surgery. Endometrial, ovarian and vulval cancers are surgically staged and therefore the surgical findings, such as nodal status, may be included in the stage. Although computed tomography (CT) and magnetic resonance imaging (MRI) may be of value in preoperative assessment, they are not included in the staging procedures. If they were included, hospitals and countries without these facilities would not be able to stage and have meaningful figures for comparison with other countries. Hence, staging is a language for allowing such comparisons and evaluating differing treatment modalities. It also helps in planning treatment and gives some indication of prognosis. In cervical cancer surgical findings, for instance, involved lymph nodes do not alter the staging but may affect management.

Treatment

Surgery is the primary treatment modality in the majority of early stage gynaecological cancers and may have an adjunctive role in more advanced cancer, such as ovarian cancer.

Reconstruction

This may be as part of primary surgery, for example at the time of vulvectomy, or may be delayed, such as after bowel resection for ovarian carcinoma.

Palliation

While there are many methods of palliation available that avoid the morbidity of surgery, there are circumstances in which the most effective long-term palliation is surgery, for instance in patients with intestinal obstruction caused by ovarian cancer. Although surgical treatment of cancer is aimed at cure and may be considered to have failed in its intent if cure is not achieved, it may provide significant palliation even in these circumstances. Palliation is considered in Chapter 14.

Complications of laparotomy

All abdominal procedures carry risk. The risks associated with surgery for cancer may be from the procedures necessary to remove the tumour or as

Table 5.1 Intraoperative complications of laparotomy

Complication	Cause
Haemorrhage	Especially from the infundibulopelvic ligaments or the bed of an incompletely resected pelvic tumour, which may require direct pressure, the use of a haemostatic substance e.g. Surgicel® (Ethicon), or even internal iliac artery ligation
Bowel damage	Due to direct tumour involvement or adhesion formation
Ureteric or bladder damage	Due to close proximity to tumour or tumour spread
Damage to large blood vessels	Compression or infiltration of external iliac arteries and veins
Direct trauma to other intra-abdominal organs	On resection of metastases or due to retraction

a direct result of the cancer itself. Intraoperative problems are detailed in Table 5.1 and postoperative complications in Table 5.2.

Ovarian carcinoma

See also Chapter 9, Ovarian cancer standards of care.

PRIMARY SURGERY

The aim of primary surgery for ovarian cancer is to confirm the diagnosis, stage the disease and remove all of the cancer or optimally cytoreduce or debulk the cancer (the amount of cancer is removed to an optimum level, which can vary).

At primary surgery, total abdominal hysterectomy, bilateral salpingo-oophorectomy, omentectomy, retroperitoneal lymph node sampling and

Table 5.2 Postoperative complications

Complication	Treatment
Ileus	Intraoperative nasogastric tube insertion is advised
Wound dehiscence or incisional hernia	Mass closure is advised
Wound infection	Give prophylactic antibiotics
Deep vein thrombosis and pulmonary embolism	Decrease risk by adequate hydration, thromboembolism-deterrent stockings, thromboprophylaxis and early mobilisation

peritoneal biopsies should be undertaken and peritoneal washings or ascitic fluid should be obtained for cytology. The surgery should usually be performed through an extended midline incision. Poor outcome in early stage ovarian cancer is often due to understaging of the disease at initial laparotomy.[1] Care must be taken to avoid intraoperative spillage that may convert stage 1a disease to stage 1c, although the prognostic significance of this is uncertain. In young women in whom the diagnosis is uncertain and who wish to retain their fertility, more conservative surgery is an option.

Germ cell tumours are relatively more common in women under 30 years of age and these can be treated with conservative surgery, enabling fertility to be retained.[2] However, young women who opt for conservative surgery at the outset must be aware that the finding of an epithelial ovarian cancer is likely to result in them requiring a further laparotomy.

For stage I disease, surgery alone results in an excellent prognosis, with a greater than 90% 5-year survival. In more advanced ovarian cancer, laparotomy and debulking of the tumour have been considered to be the mainstay of treatment since the work of Griffiths, who reported increased survival in women with residual disease of less than 1.6 cm in diameter compared with those who had bulky residual disease.[3] This has resulted in an increasing acceptance of radical surgery. There have been no randomised controlled trials comparing debulking surgery with no debulking surgery. A meta-analysis of observational studies showed that cytoreductive surgery had only a minimal effect on survival and that the major influence was the type of chemotherapy employed.[4] It has been suggested that the apparent difference in survival in patients who were optimally debulked may be a result of inherent biological characteristics, allowing complete surgical cytoreduction and at the same time enabling longer survival.[5]

Radical surgery is not without its morbidity and risks.[6] In addition, Potter et al.[7] reported on patients in whom bowel resection was undertaken to achieve optimal cytoreduction and noted poorer survival than in patients left with residual disease and not undergoing bowel resection. It is therefore appropriate that surgical cytoreduction should be performed in a gynaecological cancer centre without bowel resection unless obstruction is present or imminent. In some circumstances, primary surgery will be for relief of symptoms and diagnosis but have a minimal curative role; for instance, when bowel obstruction is present and the patient is too sick for major cytoreductive surgery.

INTERVAL SURGERY

It has been suggested that, if optimal debulking surgery is not achieved at primary surgery, a further attempt at surgery halfway through chemotherapy may improve survival. Patients with progressive disease are excluded from further surgery. A study by van der Burg demonstrated a 6-month median improvement in survival of patients undergoing interval surgery.[8] The cost–benefit of this interval procedure is not yet clear and further studies are in progress to attempt to confirm the benefits of interval surgery.

There is also currently interest in the role of timing of surgery. The diagnosis of advanced ovarian cancer can be made reliably by either CT scan and scan-guided fine-needle biopsies[9] or by open laparoscopy.[10] A number of studies have proposed chemotherapy before definitive surgery in patients with advanced ovarian carcinoma. Surwit et al.[11] reported on 29 patients and Schwartz et al.[12] described the management of 59 patients and proposed that survival was no different from a group of patients treated by primary cytoreductive surgery. Randomised prospective trials are required to establish the role of delayed primary surgery in patients with stage III ovarian carcinoma. A recent European Organisation for Research and Treatment of Cancer (EORTC) trial compared neoadjuvant chemotherapy with primary surgery for patients with stage IIIC to IV ovarian, fallopian tube and peritoneal cancer. The study concluded that neoadjuvant chemotherapy followed by cytoreduction can be considered the preferred treatment for patients with advanced ovarian cancer because neoadjuvant chemotherapy showed lower morbidity and similar survival to those patients treated with initial cytoreduction.[13]

SECOND-LOOK SURGERY

Second-look surgery has now been largely abandoned in UK practice. The aim of this surgery was to establish when chemotherapy could be stopped or alternative treatment introduced. A large prospective randomised study in 1988 showed that routine second-look laparotomy did not alter survival rates and should be abandoned.[14]

SURGERY AT RELAPSE

In the context of relapse, there is some evidence that young women who have undergone optimum primary therapy and a treatment-free interval of 12 months are more likely to have optimal second surgery with an improved median survival.[15] A significant number of women with recurrent disease will develop bowel obstruction and surgery is often the palliation method of choice.

Cervical cancer

Cervical cancer is staged clinically by means of an examination under anaesthesia, cystoscopy, sigmoidoscopy, chest X-ray and imaging of the renal tract. Increasing numbers of women are presenting with very early (stage IA) disease diagnosed at the time of a loop biopsy of the cervix and these patients may not require formal staging, provided that the disease has been completely excised. After a patient has been staged, this information is used to decide the most appropriate treatment for that individual patient.

The classification of early stage disease requires careful assessment by the pathologist and is extremely important in treatment planning (Figure 5.1).

Patients with stage IA1 can be treated by loop or cone biopsy of the cervix, thus retaining the potential for fertility. Stage IA2 can be treated by a large cone biopsy or simple hysterectomy. In this substage, however, there is an increased incidence of lymph node positivity and some would argue that if there is evidence of lymphovascular space involvement, the lymph nodes should also be removed.

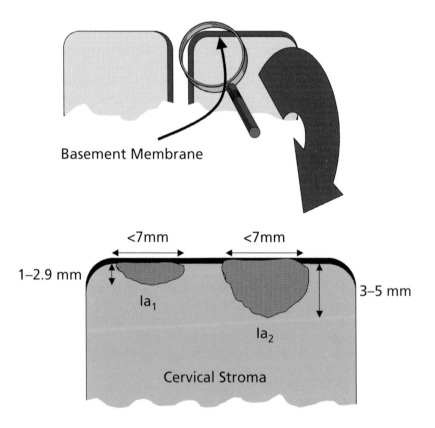

Figure 5.1 Cervical pathological substaging

Stage IB disease can be treated by surgery or radiotherapy and the surgical options are:

- radical hysterectomy with bilateral pelvic lymphadenectomy
- radical vaginal hysterectomy and laparoscopic or extraperitoneal lymph node dissection
- radical trachelectomy with laparoscopic or extraperitoneal lymph node dissection.

While these procedures are all considered therapeutic, lymph node dissection may also provide important prognostic information that is not included in staging but may demonstrate that adjuvant radiotherapy is indicated. The removal of enlarged involved lymph nodes may also have a therapeutic role, although this is not fully defined. The surgical options do allow ovarian conservation in young women. The ovaries do not need to be removed routinely in young women and the incidence of metastases in the ovary is low. However, this must be discussed with each patient individually.

Radical hysterectomy differs from a normal hysterectomy in the following ways:

- the uterine vessels are ligated close to their source
- exposure of the ureters to their insertion into the bladder
- excision of the paracervical tissues
- removal of the pelvic side wall lymph nodes
- excision of a vaginal cuff.

The possibility of radical cervical surgery with conservation of the uterine body has been pioneered in France by Dargent[16] and in the UK by Shepherd et al.[17] While there have been successful pregnancies following this form of treatment, long-term follow-up is not yet available, although early results are encouraging. In relapsed cervical cancer, radical exenterative surgery has a role for small central recurrences. However, this surgery has a high morbidity and should only be considered after multidisciplinary discussion. Only a team with the appropriate experience of this major surgery and the postoperative management of these patients should perform it. The mortality varies from 6–24% and the 5-year survival varies from 20–50%. There has also been a move towards reanastomosis of the bowel to avoid permanent colostomy and the development of continent urinary conduits.

COMPLICATIONS OF SURGICAL TREATMENT

There are some complications associated with surgical treatment of cervical cancer. These are listed in Table 5.3. Radical hysterectomy is

Table 5.3	Complications of surgical treatment of cervical cancer	
Stage	*Surgical treatment*	*Complications*
IA1	LLETZ	Secondary haemorrhage, due to infection, is treated with bed rest, antibiotics and, occasionally, cervical suturing
	Knife cone biopsy	
	Simple hysterectomy	Complications as for laparotomy
IA2	Knife cone biopsy	
	Wertheim's hysterectomy and lymph node dissection	See Table 5.4 for complications
	Radical trachelectomy	Vaginal procedure with excision of cervix, upper vagina and parametrium (uterine body is left in place). Immediate complications are infection and bleeding
IB1	Wertheim's hysterectomy and lymph node dissection	See Table 5.4 for complications
IB2	Preoperative chemoradiation and adjuvant hysterectomy	
IIA	Schauta radical vaginal hysterectomy	Involves taking a vaginal cuff, often with enlargement of the vaginal orifice with Schuchardt's incision (like a large mediolateral episiotomy). Decreased operative mortality, c.f. Wertheim's, complications as that for vaginal hysterectomy with increased risk of ureteric damage

considered a more morbid procedure than a simple hysterectomy. The complications that may occur during or following radical hysterectomy are shown in Table 5.4.

Endometrial cancer

The standard surgical management for endometrial cancer in the UK has been total abdominal hysterectomy and bilateral salpingo-oophorectomy. However, complete FIGO staging requires a full laparotomy, peritoneal washings for cytology and pelvic or para-aortic lymph node sampling. If the cervix is involved, a radical hysterectomy is required to ensure adequate excision of tumour.

While the majority of patients with endometrial carcinoma have an

Table 5.4 Complications of surgical treatment of radical hysterectomy

Complication	Cause	Comment
Haemorrhage, particularly at ureteric tunnel, paracolpos and vaginal edge, external iliac artery and vein, obturator fossa, bifurcation of common iliac artery and vein, para-aortic lymph nodes		The use of regional anaesthesia reduces small-vessel oozing
Ureteric dysfunction	Damage to the ureteric blood supply Damage to the ureteric nerve supply Oedema of the wall of the ureter Periureteric infection in the retroperitoneal space	
Ureteric stricture		Develops as a late complication and may require surgery
Ureterovaginal fistulae		Develops as a late complication and may require surgery
Bladder dysfunction	Damage to sympathetic nerves in uterosacral and cardinal ligaments results in bladder hypertonicity due to parasympathetics Oedema of bladder neck and muscle Hypotonicity as a result of overdistension of a hypertonic bladder	Catheterisation for six to eight days postoperatively is recommended
Urinary tract infection		
Vesicovaginal fistulae		
Pelvic lymphocyst at the pelvic brim or pelvic sidewall		May cause pain, obstruction or become infected. May require surgical drainage
Peripheral leg lymphoedema		May develop late and require specialised massage
Nerve damage to the obturator, genitofemoral, femoral, perineal or sciatic nerves		
Sexual dysfunction		Increased if the patient receives adjuvant radiotherapy

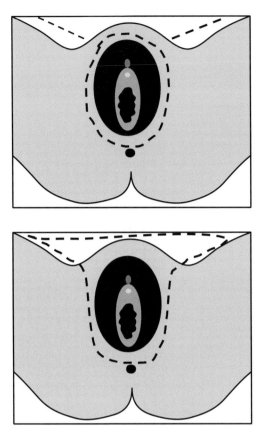

Figure 5.2 Schematic of triple incision vulvectomy and *en bloc* procedure

excellent prognosis after hysterectomy and bilateral salpingo-oophorectomy, the overall 5-year survival is only 65%.

Lymphadenectomy is indicated in cases of endometrial carcinoma in which the nodes are macroscopically enlarged. For those with no obvious nodal enlargement, the recent ASTEC study comparing lymphadenectomy with no lymphadenectomy in patients with endometrial cancer has shown no benefit from routine lymphadenectomy in these patients.[18] When fully staged surgically, 22% of patients with clinical stage I disease have extrauterine disease in the form of positive peritoneal washings, nodal disease and/or peritoneal or adnexal spread.[19] While the overall 5-year survival for patients with stage I disease is 90% and for patients with surgical stage I disease is 98%, it falls to 60% in patients with extrauterine disease.[20]

Laparoscopically assisted surgery for endometrial cancer is gaining in popularity and may decrease the morbidity and length of hospital stay for these women. The principal danger of laparoscopic surgery is the risk of injury to bowel, bladder or ureters but there have been a number of studies suggesting that this is a safe alternative.[21,22] In some women who are extremely unfit, the appropriate management may be vaginal hysterectomy.

Vulval cancer

Biopsy of a vulval lesion is essential for diagnosis before definitive surgery. This may be possible as a minor procedure under local anaesthesia or it may be performed under general anaesthesia. When performed under general anaesthesia, the operability of a lesion may be assessed, with particular reference to its proximity to the urethra or anus. Alternatively, smaller lesions may be completely excised as an excisional biopsy. Definitive surgery for vulval cancer consists of radical local excision of the vulval lesion and bilateral inguinal lymphadenectomies. Radical surgery for vulval cancer has excellent cure rates but results in high morbidity, with wound breakdown in up to 85% of patients and lymphoedema in 50% of patients. The morbidity of surgery for vulval cancer has been reduced by the introduction of the triple incision approach to replace the classical en bloc butterfly incision (Figure 5.2). This has reduced morbidity (Figures 5.3, 5.4 and 5.5) with no apparent effect on survival.[23]

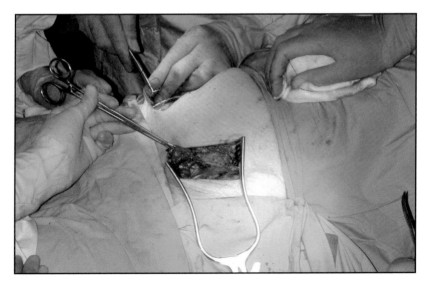

Figure 5.3 Vulval cancer separate groin incisions

The role of inguinal lymphadenectomy in vulval cancer is both diagnostic and therapeutic if the lymph nodes are involved. However, the lymph nodes are involved in only 10% of patients with vulval cancer and in 90% of cases lymphadenectomy is principally for staging and prognosis. Pelvic lymphadenectomy is no longer practised for vulval cancer. Lesions less than 1 mm depth invasion do not require inguinal lymphadenectomy and lateral lesions less than 2 cm in size can be treated by unilateral inguinal lymphadenectomy.[24] Recent studies have addressed the safety of sentinel lymph node biopsy in early vulval cancer to reduce the morbidity of treatment.[25,26] This procedure identifies a sentinel node using radioactive tracer but, as less tissue is removed, the morbidity of full groin dissection is avoided.

Surgery for vulval cancer may also involve significant reconstructive surgery, either in the form of local skin flaps (Figure 5.6) or with the aid of plastic surgeons' more advanced myocutaneous flaps using rectus abdominis or gracilis muscles. Surgery for vulval cancer may involve resection of part of the urethra or anus and urinary diversion or colostomy may be necessary. In advanced disease, the role of chemoradiotherapy before surgery should be considered to potentially preserve pelvic anatomy.

SURGERY IN RECURRENT OR ADVANCED DISEASE

Surgery may have a palliative or curative role in advanced or recurrent disease. Women with localised recurrent disease in the pelvis or abdomen

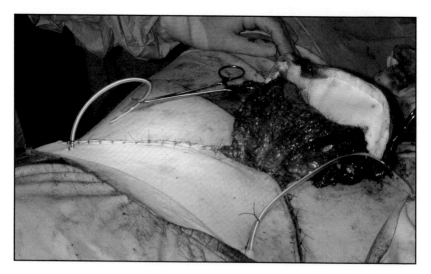

Figure 5.4 En bloc radical vulvectomy

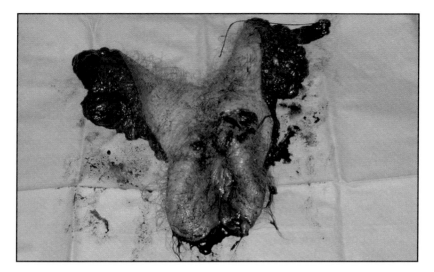

Figure 5.5 En bloc radical vulvectomy specimen

may be suitable for surgical management. This may involve cooperation with colorectal surgeons, urologists or vascular surgeons. Patients should be carefully assessed preoperatively to exclude distant metastases and to establish the potential for curative treatment.

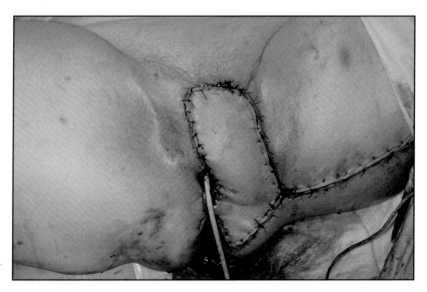

Figure 5.6 Simple rotational flap

References

1. Venesmaa P. Epithelial ovarian cancer: impact of surgery and chemotherapy on survival during 1977–1990. *Obstet Gynecol* 1994;84:8–11.

2. Abu-Rustum N, Aghajanian C. Management of malignant germ cell tumours of the ovary. *Semin Oncol* 1998;25:235–42.

3. Griffiths CT. Surgical resection of tumour bulk in the primary treatment of ovarian carcinoma. *Natl Cancer Inst Monogr* 1975;42:101–4.

4. Hunter RW, Alexander NDE, Soutter WP. Meta-analysis of surgery in advanced ovarian carcinoma: is cytoreduction an independent determinant of prognosis? *Am J Obstet Gynecol* 1992;166:504–11.

5. Hoskins WJ, McGuire WP, Brady MF, Homesly HD, Creasman WT, Berman M, *et al*. The effects of diameter of largest residual disease on survival after primary cytoreductive surgery in patients with suboptimal residual ovarian carcinoma. *Am J Obstet Gynecol* 1994;170:974–80.

6. Guidozzi F, Ball JHS. Extensive primary cytoreductive surgery for advanced epithelial ovarian cancer. *Gynecol Oncol* 1994;53:326–30.

7. Potter ME, Partridge EE, Hatch KD, Soong SJ, Austin JM, Shingleton HM. Primary surgical therapy of ovarian cancer: how much and when. *Gynecol Oncol* 1991;40:195–200.

8. Van der Burg ME, van Lent M, Buyse M, Kobierska A, Colombo N, Favalli G, *et al*. The effect of debulking surgery after induction chemotherapy on the prognosis in advanced epithelial ovarian cancer. *N Engl J Med* 1995;332:629–34.

9. Nelson BE, Rosenfield AT, Schwartz PE. Pre-operative abdominopelvic computed tomographic prediction of optimal cytoreduction in epithelial ovarian carcinoma. *J Clin Oncol* 1993;11:166–72.

10. Van Dam PA, Decloedt J, Tjama W, Vergote 1b. Diagnostic laparoscopy to assess operability of advanced ovarian cancer: a feasibility study. *Eur J Gynaecol Oncol* 1997;18:272–3.

11. Surwit E, Childers J, Atlas M, Nour M, Hatch K, Hallam A, *et al*. Neoadjuvant chemotherapy for advanced ovarian cancer. *Int J Gynecol Cancer* 1996;6:356–61.

12. Schwartz PE, Chambers JT, Makuch R. Neoadjuvant chemotherapy for advanced ovarian cancer. *Gynecol Oncol* 1994;53:33–7.

13 Vergote I, Trape CG, Amant F, Kristensen GB, Sandi JE, Ehler T, *et al*. EORTC-GCG/NCI-CTG randomised trial comparing primary debulking surgery with neoadjuvant chemotherapy in stage 3–4 ovarian, fallopian tube and peritoneal cancer. OVCA 12th Biennial Meeting, International Gynaecological Cancer Society, Oct 25–28, Bangkok 2008.

14. Luesley D, Lawton F, Blackledge G, Hilton C, Kelly R, Rollason T, *et al*. Failure of second-look laparotomy to influence survival in epithelial ovarian cancer. *Lancet* 1988;ii:599–603.

15. Segna RA, Dottino PR, Mandeli JP, Konsker K, Cohen CJ, *et al*. Secondary cytoreduction for ovarian cancer following cisplatin therapy. *J Clin Oncol* 1993;11:434–9.

16. Dargent D. Laparoscopic surgery and gynaecologic cancer. *Curr Opin Obstet Gynecol* 1993;5:294–300.

17. Shepherd JH, Crawford RAF, Oram DH. Radical trachelectomy: a way to preserve fertility in the treatment of early cervical cancer. *Br J Obstet Gynaecol* 1998;105:912–16.

18. ASTEC Study Group. Efficacy of systematic lymphadenectomy in endometrial cancer. *Lancet* 2009;373:125–36.

19. Creasman WT, Morrow CP, Bundy BN, Homeseley HD, Graham JE, Heller PB. Surgical pathologic spread patterns of endometrial cancer. A Gynaecologic Oncology Cancer Group Study. *Cancer* 1987;60:2035–41.

20. Gal D, Recio FO, Zamurovic D. The New International Federation of Obstetrics and Gynecology surgical staging and survival rates in early endometrial carcinoma. *Cancer* 1992;69:200–2.

21. Holub Z, Voracek J, Shomani A. A comparison of laparoscopic surgery with an open procedure in endometrial cancer. *Eur J Gynaecol Oncol* 1998;19:294–6.

22. Spirtos NM, Schlaerth JB, Gross GM, Spirtos TW, Schlaerth AC, Ballon SC. Cost and quality-of-life analyses of surgery for early endometrial cancer: laparotomy versus laparoscopy. *Am J Obstet Gynecol* 1996;174:1795–9.

23. Hacker NF, Leuchter RS, Berek JS, Castaldo TW, Lagasse LD. Radical vulvectomy and bilateral inguinal lymphadenectomy through separate groin incisions. *Obstet Gynecol* 1981;58:574–9.

24. Cavanagh D, Hoffman MS. Controversies in the management of vulvar cancer. *Br J Obstet Gynaecol* 1996;103:293–300.

25. Van Der Zee AG, Oonk MH, De Hullu JA, Ansink AC, Vergote I, Verheijen RH, *et al*. Sentinel node dissection is safe in the treatment of early stage vulvar cancer. *J Clin Oncol* 2008;26:884–9.

26. Hampl M, Hantsschmann P, Michels W, Hillemanns P. Validation of the accuracy of the sentinel node procedure in patients with vulvar cancer. Results of a multicentre study in Germany. *Gynecol Oncol* 2008;111:282–8.

6 Role of laparoscopic surgery

Introduction

The first decade of the 21st century has seen minimal access surgery in oncology progress from simple laparoscopically assisted vaginal procedures to complex operations such as radical hysterectomy and lymph node dissection. Laparoscopic surgery is associated with reduced levels of postoperative pain, early discharge from hospital and an earlier return to normal activity. However, many surgeons have been reluctant to replace abdominal radical surgery with laparoscopic surgery because of concerns that it does not replicate the radicalism of open surgery. In 1987, Dargent reported combining a radical vaginal hysterectomy with a laparoscopic pelvic lymph node dissection in the management of cervical cancer.[1] Following this, a number of reports have been published on the feasibility and safety of laparoscopic surgery in treating gynaecological cancer. More recently, new energy modalities, such as the argon beam coagulator and the harmonic scalpel, have allowed safe dissection of tissue with minimal thermal spread to nearby structures.

Cervical cancer

The management of cervical cancer is based on the extent of disease spread using the FIGO staging system. This is based on clinical examination and limited radiological assessment. Clinical staging allows only limited assessment of the nodal status, which is considered one of the most important prognostic factors.

FIGO stage IA1 cancers have a minimal risk of spread into the surrounding parametrium and the pelvic lymph nodes. In the UK, these cancers are treated by local excision methods such as cone biopsy or large-loop excision of the transformation zone (LLETZ). Assuming that the margins are free of malignancy and dysplasia, these local procedures are considered optimal. Older women with coexisting gynaecological problems may wish to consider a vaginal hysterectomy once more advanced disease has been ruled out. In other countries, women with stage IA1 disease with extensive lymphovascular space involvement may be offered a pelvic node dissection combined with local excision or a simple hysterectomy.

The surgical management of women with FIGO stage IA2 or IB1 squamous or adenocarcinoma of the cervix is a radical hysterectomy and pelvic lymph node dissection. Women with large diameter tumours (greater than 4 cm), such as FIGO stage IB2 tumour, are at high risk of requiring postoperative chemoradiotherapy and so are not generally offered laparoscopic surgery. This because it may be difficult to obtain a clear surgical margins at radical resection and the high risk of microscopic spread into the parametrium and to the pelvic lymph nodes. Preoperative magnetic resonance assessment can accurately determine tumour volume and depth of invasion into the cervical stroma.[2]

The concept of sentinel node detection is appealing in the laparoscopic management of cervical cancer. The sentinel lymph node is the first lymph node reached by metastasising cancer cells from a tumour. Laparoscopic removal of the sentinel node rather than a full node dissection would reduce the risk of lower limb lymphoedema. If the sentinel node were positive then the woman would be given chemoradiotherapy rather than undergoing unnecessary surgery and then chemoradiotherapy. This would reduce the extra complications arising from using both treatment modalities. Most research studies have used a combination of intracervical injections of patent blue dye to aid laparoscopic lymphatic channel visualisation and technetium-99 isotope to allow precise location of the sentinel node with a gamma probe or Geiger counter.[3] To date, sentinel node removal has not replaced full nodal pending the publication of continuing studies.

Chemoradiotherapy is considered the main treatment for advanced cervical cancers such as FIGO stage II and above. The standard radiotherapy fields avoid the para-aortic region because of the high risk of small bowel toxicity. The risk of para-aortic node metastases increases with tumour stage, volume and positive pelvic lymph nodes. The reported incidence of positive para-aortic nodes in stage II disease is 12–19% and in stage III is 29–33%.[4] Both computed tomography and positron emission tomography are poor at detecting micrometastases to the para-aortic nodes in cervical cancer.[5,6] Dissection by laparotomy results in delaying the administration of chemoradiotherapy and increases toxicity from adhesion formation. Laparoscopy results in less adhesion than laparotomy. The extraperitoneal route is associated with lower rates of adhesion formation than conventional transperitoneal laparoscopy in porcine models.[7]

It is possible to perform exenterative procedures for a central recurrence of cervical cancer using a laparoscopically assisted approach.[8] A combination of the level of expertise required, length of operating time and the small number of women requiring this operation means that this procedure will be confined to extremely specialised centres in the foreseeable future.

Endometrial cancer

The majority of women with endometrial cancer will be cured by a total hysterectomy and bilateral salpingo-oophorectomy. The results of the ASTEC study (A Study in the Treatment of Endometrial Cancer) suggest that there is no benefit in performing a pelvic lymphadenopathy in early cancers.[9] A meta-analysis has reported lower complication rates and similar recurrence and survival after laparoscopic surgery.[10] Many of the women with endometrioid cancers are obese and ideally suited to benefit from laparoscopic surgery with smaller wounds, lower infection rates and early mobilisation. The main limiting step would appear to be the ability of the woman to tolerate anaesthesia, especially in the head-down position, and its resulting effect on respiratory function. Women with some degree of uterovaginal prolapse are candidates for a laparoscopically assisted vaginal hysterectomy, combined with removal of the ovaries and pelvic washings. Many women who are obese will have minimal prolapse and limited vaginal access. These women are frequently suitable for a total laparoscopic hysterectomy using a gas-tight vaginal tube.

Women with type-II endometrial cancer, such as serous adenocarcinoma, have a very high risk of spread beyond the uterus, even with limited gross myometrial invasion. A limited number of these women were included in the ASTEC study and many oncology centres will still perform full surgical staging, including hysterectomy, bilateral salpingo-oophorectomy, pelvic and para-aortic node dissection. The cephalic extent of the para-aortic node dissection is traditionally to the level of the inferior mesenteric artery. This can be performed laparoscopically either via a transperitoneal or extra peritoneal route.

Ovarian cancer

Laparoscopy is frequently used in the management of adnexal masses by gynaecologists. A number of benign gynaecological conditions result in a raised serum CA125, such as endometriosis and fibroids. Imaging can aid in differentiating between benign and malignant adnexal masses. Radiological features suggestive of cancer include multiloculated cysts, solid areas, internal septation, papillary projections and ascites.

Ovarian cysts or masses can be assessed for the possibility of cancer by risk of malignancy index.[11,12] These commonly combine menopausal status of the women, serum CA125 level and the ultrasonographical or radiological features of the lesion. They have a sensitivity of 71–80% and specificity of 92–96%. The risk of malignancy indices are less likely to identify a stage I ovarian cancer as abnormal because 50% will have a normal serum CA125 level. Approximately 30% of women with ovarian cancers apparently confined to the ovaries will be upstaged by a gynaecological oncologist.[13]

This is important for a number of reasons: it may influence whether or not chemotherapy is given, it may result in complete debulking of the cancer and determining the true prognosis. It is difficult to predict which women with ovarian masses will require full surgical staging. A pragmatic approach in young women with complex ovarian masses involves the removal of adnexal masses intact in a sealed bag, combined with performance of pelvic washings and careful inspection of the abdominal cavity. Postoperatively, those women with confirmed malignancy can be offered staging if this will affect the treatment or prognosis.

In older women with complex masses or those considered to have a high risk of cancer, an intraoperative frozen section histopathological analysis can be performed. A study from the Gateshead Gynaecological Oncology Centre reported a sensitivity of 92%, specificity of 88%, positive predictive value of 82% and negative predictive value of 95% for frozen section analysis.[14] This is equally important in determining which women should not be exposed to unnecessary surgery such as a para-aortic node dissection.

Staging requires resection of adnexa, pelvic cytology, infracolic omentectomy, peritoneal biopsies, appendicectomy (in the case of mucinous tumours) and pelvic and para-aortic lymph node dissection. Laparoscopic staging is possible, though requires a high degree of specialist training. Several centres have reported on full laparoscopic staging and have found it feasible.[15–17] A case–control study comparing staging via laparoscopy or laparotomy in 80 women found no difference in specimen sizes and lymph nodal counts.[18] The laparoscopic group had reduced levels of blood loss and a reduced hospital stay.

The role of laparoscopy in advanced stage ovarian cancer is controversial. Laparoscopy can be used to obtain biopsies if the origin of the tumour is in doubt but this can normally be performed by radiological directed biopsies. Laparoscopy does have the advantage of assessing the potential for optimal debulking surgery to minimal residual disease. This indication is of unproven benefit and is infrequently performed outside clinical trials. Laparoscopy in advanced disease has the potential to produce serious harm, including bowel injury and port site metastases.

Surgical techniques

RADICAL HYSTERECTOMY

A radical hysterectomy may be performed as a laparoscopically assisted procedure or as a total laparoscopic procedure. The type of operation depends on the woman's degree of uterovaginal prolapse, vaginal access and the ability of the surgeon to perform dissection of the ureteric tunnel via the vagina.

Complications include haemorrhage, damage to bowel, bladder, ureter and autonomic nerve dysfunction. A learning curve is apparent, with complication rates decreasing over time. A case series of 295 women reported an operating time of 162 minutes including pelvic lymph node dissection and conversion to laparotomy in five women due to bleeding or bowel injury. No randomised controlled trials have been published comparing laparoscopic with open abdominal radical hysterectomy. Several retrospective studies have reported that laparoscopic surgery is safe and offers outcomes equivalent to open surgery. These studies suggest longer operating times, reduced rates of bleeding and similar rates of other complications.[19] One study compared laparoscopy with open radical hysterectomy. The recurrence rate was 14% compared with 12% and the mortality rate 10% compared with 8% over a median follow-up period of 26 months.[20]

Technique

The woman is placed in the modified lithotomy position using laparoscopy boots to allow intraoperative leg manipulation. The woman's arms are tucked in at her sides to avoid prolonged traction on her brachial plexus. An indwelling urinary catheter should be inserted prior to laparoscopy and antibiotic prophylaxis administered. An 11-mm port is generally placed in the umbilicus with a further port in the suprapubic region and two 5-mm ports in the lateral lower quadrant, lateral to the inferior epigastric vessels. The retroperitoneal space is opened by transecting the round ligaments at the level of the obliterated umbilical artery and continuing the incision cephalad to allow identification of the ureter where it crosses the iliac vessels. Any suspicious lymph nodes should be sent for frozen section analysis. If results are positive then the operation should be abandoned and chemoradiotherapy considered as primary therapy.

The paravesical space is opened by dissecting the tissue lateral to the obliterated umbilical artery down to the pelvic floor. This then allows the space medial to the artery to be opened. Dissecting between the ureter and the internal iliac vessels opens the pararectal space; this is followed by separation of the ureter from the peritoneal attachments. Once the spaces are opened, the uterine vessels are found by following the umbilical artery cephalad (Figure 6.1). The vessels are transected at their origin. The ovaries are rarely a site of metastatic spread in cervical cancer and can be conserved.

Surgeons trained in radical vaginal hysterectomy may wish to transfer to the vaginal part of the operation. This involves circumscribing the vagina around the cervix and dissecting the bladder off the vagina and opening the rectovaginal space. The bladder pillars are then isolated and the ureter identified and the pillar divided. Once the uterosacral ligaments are divided the uterus can be removed.

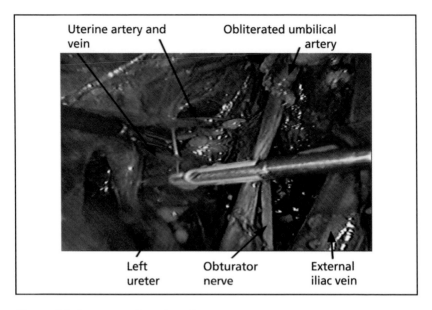

Figure 6.1 Demonstration of uterine artery

For a total laparoscopic procedure, the visceral peritoneum at the interface of the bladder and cervix is cut. The uterus is manipulated into neutral position and pushed cephalad to help dissection of the bladder off the cervix and vagina to allow a vaginal cuff. The rectovaginal space is developed and the peritoneum over the uterosacral ligaments is transected.

The parametrium is drawn over the ureter by the assistant on the contralateral side from the ureter. The magnification of the laparoscope allows the surgeon to seal the small vessels in the ureteric tunnel that normally cause troublesome bleeding during open surgery. At this stage, the surgeon is operating directly on top of the ureter and energy sources such as the harmonic scalpel and argon beam coagulator may allow more precise dissection compared with conventional bipolar diathermy. The ureters are dissected and mobilised to their insertion into the bladder. The uterosacral ligaments are divided and a hollow vaginal tube inserted. The tube delineates the vagina and provides a gas tight seal. The vagina is circumscribed around the tube and the uterus is removed via the vagina. The vault may at this stage be sutured vaginally or laparoscopically from above. The woman can generally be discharged within 24–48 hours of surgery, returning after 72 hours for a trial of urinary catheter removal and post-void ultrasound scan.

PELVIC LYMPH NODE DISSECTION

The main indication for a pelvic lymph node dissection is in the management of cervical cancer often combined with radical surgery. Following the publication of the ASTEC study, the need for pelvic node dissection in endometrial cancer has been questioned.[9] In early ovarian cancer, a full staging procedure should include at least a unilateral pelvic lymph node dissection and para-aortic nodes dissection to determine the need for adjuvant chemotherapy and detail prognostic information.

The number of lymph nodes removed is comparable to open pelvic node dissection. The main disadvantage is the increase in the operating time required, although this decreases with the experience of the surgeon. Advantages include a reduction in bleeding from small vessels owing to the pressure of the pneumoperitoneum. The rate of blood transfusion is lower for laparoscopic surgery than open dissection.[21] The superior view afforded by the laparoscope should decrease the risk of injury to vessels in the obturator fossa. The rates of other complications such as injury to the ureter, nerves and the formation of lymphocyst are similar to open surgery.[22]

Technique

The woman is placed in a similar position to that described above for a laparoscopic radical hysterectomy. Pelvic lymph node dissection is normally performed with another procedure, such as hysterectomy, and this may influence the placement and the size of ports used. The dissected nodes can be removed through an 11/12-mm suprapubic port or via the vagina if a hysterectomy is performed. To move the small bowel out of the operative site, the women is placed in the Trendelenberg position. The assistant grasps the round ligament and the peritoneum is opened at the level of the external iliac vessels. The incision is extended parallel to the infundibulopelvic ligament to the psoas muscle. The sigmoid is mobilised out of the operative field on the left. The external iliac vessels are identified followed by the ureter then and internal iliac artery. The genitofemoral nerve running the medial margin of the psoas muscle should be preserved. The lymphatic fat pad overlying the psoas and iliac vessels is grasped and dissected off in the longitudinal manner with the aim of entering the bloodless adventitial layer. The nodal tissue, from midway along the common iliac vessels down to the caudal level of the deep circumflex vein crossing over the external iliac artery, is removed. This should include all nodal tissue between the artery and vein and the psoas muscle along the medial level of the internal iliac artery.

The next stage of the procedure is to remove the nodes in the obturator fossa. The obturator nerve should be identified and guarded before any sharp dissection. The nodes should be swept away from the nerve with careful attention paid to the area below the nerve to avoid damage to the numerous vessels present in this area. The ideal scenario is to remove the node in a single nodal unit to reduce the risk of nodal fracture leading to tumour dissemination and port site metastases.

LAPAROSCOPIC EXTRAPERITONEAL PARA-AORTIC NODE DISSECTION

There is limited evidence concerning the impact laparoscopic para-aortic nodal dissection has on survival in advanced cervical cancer. A single study to date has reported that women with positive laparoscopically resected para-aortic nodes have the same overall survival as women with para-aortic negative nodes.[23] Both transperitoneal and extraperitoneal para-aortic node counts are similar to those found in open surgery.[22]

Potential complications include haemorrhage, ureteric damage and lymphocyst formation. The rate of complication is related to the experience of the surgeons involved and the learning curve appears to be steep compared with other operations such as radical hysterectomy. In a series of 184 women, the intraoperative haemorrhage rate was 2.2% and all cases were controlled by laparoscopic clipping without the need for laparotomy.[24] The median operating time was 155 minutes and the median time to discharge was 1.4 days. It is interesting to note that laparoscopic para-aortic dissection can safely be performed as day surgery.[25]

Technique

The woman is placed in the standard supine position after urinary catheterisation and both legs are deviated to the right side of the operating table to increase the space between the bony pelvis and thoracic cage on the left side. The transperitoneal laparoscopy is carried out to exclude carcinomatosis and assess the ovaries. A 1.5–2-cm incision is made 3 cm medial to the left anterior superior iliac spine. This incision is carried through the skin, fat and anterior abdominal wall muscles without opening the peritoneum. Under the visual guidance of the transperitoneal laparoscope, a finger is place in extraperitoneal space and careful blunt finger dissection is carried out. To create the extraperitoneal space, the peritoneum is pushed off the abdominal wall until the psoas muscle and the external iliac artery are felt. A port is inserted under finger guidance in the mid-maxillary line and a balloon tracer placed in the original incision site to seal the site. The space is inflated with carbon dioxide gas to maximum pressure of 12 mmHg. The camera is placed through the balloon trocar and a further trocar placed in the anterior axillary line.

The left ureter, ovarian and common iliac vessels are indentified and the ureter is elevated while still attached to the peritoneum, producing a bow-like effect. Key structures to be identified are the inferior mesenteric artery, vena cava, right ovarian vessel and right ureter. If the dissection is to be carried above the inferior mesenteric artery, the insertion of the left ovarian vein into the left renal vein needs to be identified through careful dissection (Figure 6.2).

A systematic dissection of the lymph nodes should be performed from midway along the left common iliac arteries to the inferior mesenteric artery and over the presacral region, with careful attention paid to the middle sacral vessels and the iliac veins. The dissection should move over to the right side with the removal of aortocaval nodes and the caval nodes, with coagulation of perforating vessels such as the Fellow's vein. It can be difficult to obtain an optimal view of the right side of the vena cava. The dissection may continue up the renal veins at the point of the ovarian vein insertion into the vena cava and the left renal vein. The lymph nodes are removed through the larger port and haemostasis checked. The procedure is completed with marsupialisation or opening of the peritoneum over the left pelvic gutter under transperitoneal guidance to reduce the incidence of postoperative lymphocyst formation.

Potential immediate complications include haemorrhage, ureteric damage and bowel injury. The majority of vascular injuries can be treated with a combination of compression with swabs and bipolar diathermy. Frequently, the tamponade effect afforded by the carbon dioxide in a confined space at pressures of around 12 mmHg limits all but major bleeding. The incidence of symptomatic lymphocele is significantly

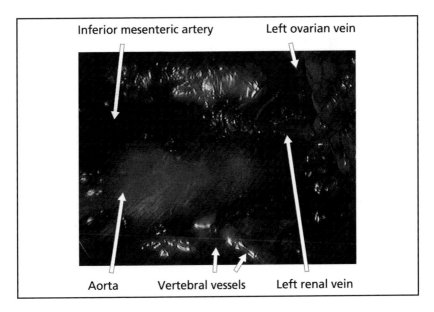

Figure 6.2 Aorta following nodal dissection

reduced by the marsupialisation of the peritoneum at the end of the operation.[26]

KEY POINTS

- Gynaecological oncology in the UK has been slow to embrace laparoscopic surgery because of concerns that it may not replicate the radicalism of open surgery.
- These concerns have been addressed in publications from major gynaecological oncology centres throughout the world.
- Laparoscopic surgery has now become an essential part of training in gynaecological oncology programmes.
- Energy modalities such as the argon beam coagulator and the harmonic scalpel have allowed safe dissection of tissue with minimal thermal spread to nearby structures.
- New developments such as robotic laparoscopic surgery and the use of small single-site incisions are likely to further expand the number of women suitable for laparoscopic management and reduce morbidity.

References

1. Dargent D, Mathevet P. Schauta's vaginal hysterectomy combined with laparoscopic lymphadenectomy. *Baillieres Clin Obstet Gynaecol* 1995;9:691–705.

2. Hricak H, Gatsonis C, Coakley FV, Snyder B, Reinhold C, Schwartz LH, *et al*. Early invasive cervical cancer: CT and MR imaging in preoperative evaluation: ACRIN/GOG comparative study of diagnostic performance and interobserver variability. *Radiology* 2007;245:491–8.

3. Abu-Rustum NR, Khoury-Collado F, Gemignani ML. Techniques of sentinel lymph node identification for early-stage cervical and uterine cancer. *Gynecol Oncol* 2008;111(2 Suppl):S44–50.

4. DeVita VT, Hellman S, Rosenberg SA. *Cancer : Principles and Practice of Oncology*. 3rd ed. Philadelphia, PA: Lippincott; 1989.

5. Loft A, Berthelsen AK, Roed H, Ottosen C, Lundvall L, Knudsen J, *et al*. The diagnostic value of PET/CT scanning in patients with cervical cancer: a prospective study. *Gynecol Oncol* 2007;106:29–34.

6. Sironi S, Buda A, Picchio M, Perego P, Moreni R, Pellegrino A, *et al*. Lymph node metastasis in patients with clinical early-stage cervical cancer: detection with integrated FDG PET/CT. *Radiology* 2006;238:272–9.

7. Lanvin D, Elhage A, Henry B, Leblanc E, Querleu D, Delobelle-Deroide A. Accuracy and safety of laparoscopic lymphadenectomy: an experimental prospective randomized study. *Gynecol Oncol* 1997;67:83–7.

8. Ferron G, Lim TY, Pomel C, Soulie M, Querleu D. Creation of the miami pouch during laparoscopic-assisted pelvic exenteration: the initial experience. *Int J Gynecol Cancer* 2009;19:466–70.

9. Kitchener H, Swart AM, Qian Q, Amos C, Parmar MK. Efficacy of systematic pelvic lymphadenectomy in endometrial cancer (MRC ASTEC trial): a randomised study. *Lancet* 2009;373:125–36.

10. Ju W, Myung SK, Kim Y, Choi HJ, Kim SC. Comparison of laparoscopy and laparotomy for management of endometrial carcinoma: a meta-analysis. *Int J Gynecol Cancer* 2009;19:400–6.

11. Jacobs I, Oram D, Fairbanks J, Turner J, Frost C, Grudzinskas JG. A risk of malignancy index incorporating CA 125, ultrasound and menopausal status for the accurate preoperative diagnosis of ovarian cancer. *Br J Obstet Gynaecol* 1990;97:922–9.

12. Tingulstad S, Hagen B, Skjeldestad FE, Halvorsen T, Nustad K, Onsrud M. The risk-of-malignancy index to evaluate potential ovarian cancers in local hospitals. *Obstet Gynecol* 1999;93:448–52.

13. Young RC, Decker DG, Wharton JT, Piver MS, Sindelar WF, Edwards BK, *et al.* Staging laparotomy in early ovarian cancer. *JAMA* 1983;250:3072–6.

14. Naik R, Cross P, Lopes A, Godfrey K, Hatem MH. 'True' versus 'apparent' stage 1 epithelial ovarian cancer: value of frozen section analysis. *Int J Gynecol Cancer* 2006;16(Suppl 1):41–6.

15. Childers JM, Lang J, Surwit EA, Hatch KD. Laparoscopic surgical staging of ovarian cancer. *Gynecol Oncol* 1995;59:25–33.

16. Tozzi R, Kohler C, Ferrara A, Schneider A. Laparoscopic treatment of early ovarian cancer: surgical and survival outcomes. *Gynecol Oncol* 2004;93:199–203.

17. Leblanc E, Querleu D, Narducci F, Occelli B, Papageorgiou T, Sonoda Y. Laparoscopic restaging of early stage invasive adnexal tumors: a 10-year experience. *Gynecol Oncol* 2004;94:624–9.

18. Chi DS, Abu-Rustum NR, Sonoda Y, Ivy J, Rhee E, Moore K, *et al.* The safety and efficacy of laparoscopic surgical staging of apparent stage 1 ovarian and fallopian tube cancers. *Am J Obstet Gynecol* 2005;192:1614–19.

19. Frumovitz M, dos Reis R, Sun CC, Milam MR, Bevers MW, Brown J, *et al.* Comparison of total laparoscopic and abdominal radical hysterectomy for patients with early-stage cervical cancer. *Obstet Gynecol* 2007;110:96–102.

20. Li G, Yan X, Shang H, Wang G, Chen L, Han Y. A comparison of laparoscopic radical hysterectomy and pelvic lymphadenectomy and laparotomy in the treatment of Ib–2a cervical cancer. *Gynecol Oncol* 2007;105:176–80.

21. Scribner DR Jr, Walker JL, Johnson GA, McMeekin SD, Gold MA, Mannel RS. Surgical management of early-stage endometrial cancer in the elderly: is laparoscopy feasible? *Gynecol Oncol* 2001;83:563–8.

22. Querleu D, Leblanc E, Cartron G, Narducci F, Ferron G, Martel P. Audit of preoperative and early complications of laparoscopic lymph node dissection in 1000 gynecologic cancer patients. *Am J Obstet Gynecol* 2006;195:1287–92.

23. Marnitz S, Kohler C, Roth C, Fuller J, Hinkelbein W, Schneider A. Is there a benefit of pretreatment laparoscopic transperitoneal surgical staging in patients with advanced cervical cancer? *Gynecol Oncol* 2005;99:536–44.

24. Leblanc E, Narducci F, Frumovitz M, Lesoin A, Castelain B, Baranzelli MC, *et al.* Therapeutic value of pretherapeutic extraperitoneal laparoscopic staging of locally advanced cervical carcinoma. *Gynecol Oncol* 2007;105:304–11.

25. Tillmanns T, Lowe MP. Safety, feasibility, and costs of outpatient laparoscopic extraperitoneal aortic nodal dissection for locally advanced cervical carcinoma. *Gynecol Oncol* 2007;106:370–4.

26. Sonoda Y, Leblanc E, Querleu D, Castelain B, Papageorgiou TH, Lambaudie E, *et al.* Prospective evaluation of surgical staging of advanced cervical cancer via a laparoscopic extraperitoneal approach. *Gynecol Oncol* 2003;91:326–31.

7 Radiotherapy: principles and applications

Introduction

The therapeutic use of radiation in gynaecological cancer quickly followed the discovery of X-rays by Roentgen in 1895 and radium by the Curies in 1898. The aim of radiotherapy is to destroy the cancer if possible without damaging the surrounding normal tissues. The application of a cancericidal dose of radiation to the cancer must be balanced against the inevitable collateral damage caused to local normal organs at risk. Radiotherapy treatment can involve a combination of external beam radiotherapy and brachytherapy. External radiotherapy (teletherapy) employs the use of a high-energy photon (X-ray) beam generated from a linear accelerator. Brachytherapy (Greek *brachy*, short) involves the use of sealed radiotherapy sources placed close to the treated tissue. The sources may be placed in the natural cavities of the vagina or uterus (intracavitary treatment) or needles or tubes inserted into the tissues (interstitial brachytherapy). The two modalities of external beam radiotherapy and brachytherapy can be combined or used individually.

Radiobiology

Radiotherapy uses the damaging effects of ionising radiation on cellular DNA. X-rays and, less commonly, gamma-rays are the commonly used forms of ionising radiation. The 'four Rs' form the basis of radiobiology: repair, repopulation, reoxygenation and redistribution.[1]

Cancer cells and normal tissue cells vary in their ability to repair the damage caused by radiation. This difference can be exploited by dividing up (fractionating) the dose of radiotherapy to increase the lethal damage to tumour cells, while allowing normal tissues to repair.

During radiotherapy, viable cells will continue to divide. This is the process of repopulation. A course of radiotherapy must kill not only the original tumour cells but also those formed by repopulation during the treatment period.

Well-oxygenated cells are more sensitive to radiation-induced damage than hypoxic cells. Reoxygenation is the process whereby relatively hypoxic areas acquire the perfusion left by the more radiosensitive, well-oxygenated cells that have been killed by previous fractions of radiotherapy.

Cells vary in their response to the effects of radiotherapy throughout the cell cycle. Cells in the G1, early S and G2/M phases are highly sensitive, whereas cells in the late S phase are relatively resistant. Fractionation of the radiotherapy exploits this redistribution of cells through the stages of the cell cycle.

Planning

Radiotherapy planning involves three-dimensional localisation of the treatment volume and assessment of the surrounding normal tissues. The patient has a CT planning scan (see chapter 4). The clinician draws the target volumes and organs at risk on a planning computer. The planning process outlines the tissues to be treated. The target volume is the demonstrable cancer and any tissues at risk of containing cancer. The principal organs at risk for most gynaecological cancers are the bladder and rectum. A three-dimensional model of the target volume and organs at risk is displayed by the planning department. From that model, a treatment plan showing an isodose distribution is developed, using multiple radiation fields and shielding of normal tissue by multileaf collimators or lead blocks. Inevitably, the bowel and bladder will also receive some radiation but it is the 'art' of radiotherapy to plan the beams so that the tumour receives a cancericidal dose while the normal tissue doses remain within tolerance. Tattoos are placed on the patient to aid accurate positioning for each fraction of radiotherapy.

Implementation of brachytherapy

Brachytherapy has the advantage of delivering a high dose in the proximity of the sources while limiting the dose to normal tissues. Various intracavity systems have been designed. The 'live' systems as originally developed in Paris, Stockholm, Manchester and Sheffield have now been replaced in most of the world by afterloading equipment. Live brachytherapy exposes the operating doctor, the theatre staff and the ward nurses to the risks of radiation throughout the period in which the patient is being treated.

Afterloading systems are mechanical devices that load the actual radioactive sources into the patient remotely once she is on the ward in a protected room. The operating doctor merely inserts non-radioactive tubes in the correct arrangement and the afterloading apparatus is connected to these tubes later. This system protects the staff at the time of insertion and on the ward. It also allows more time for the radiotherapist to adjust the insertion to ensure the best arrangement to treat the patient and for more flexibility in the arrangement of sources. The most common mechanical afterloading system is the Selectron. The high dose rate Selectron allows the dose to be delivered in minutes and thus on an outpatient basis.

IMPORTANCE OF RECTAL AND BLADDER DOSES

The limiting tissues for gynaecological brachytherapy are the rectum and bladder. The tolerances for these tissues were empirically derived. The dose rate to the rectum is reduced by the mechanical spacing imposed by the applicators themselves, any packing inserted by the operating doctor and any inbuilt shielding.

DOSE PRESCRIPTION FOR RADIOTHERAPY IN CARCINOMA OF THE CERVIX

The doses of radiotherapy employed in treating carcinoma of the cervix depend particularly on the intracavitary technique and equipment used. The doses are prescribed at conventional Manchester Points A and B. Point A is defined as 2 cm lateral to the midline and 2 cm above the lateral vaginal fornix. Point B is 3 cm lateral to Point A. With combined external and intracavity brachytherapy most clinicians would aim for a combined total dose of 70–80 Gy at Point A and 50–60 Gy to Point B. The balance of the contribution of external and internal radiotherapy used to achieve these doses depends on the individual configuration of the patient's cancer, and the particular technique and equipment favoured by the clinicians.

The design of radiotherapy for carcinoma of the cervix depends on the extent of the cancer. In general higher stage cancers are given more of the dose from external beam and less from the brachytherapy. Apart from very early cancers it is usual to give the external beam radiotherapy first. This allows the cancer to shrink so that the anatomical arrangement of the brachytherapy improves.

Adverse effects of radiotherapy

The radiation tolerance of normal tissues is related to the acute or chronic radiation reactions that occur in them. The acceptable tolerances determine the way in which radiotherapy is planned. Tolerance is a relative term in that we will accept a greater degree of damage to normal tissues if the aim is radical rather than palliative.

The acute reaction encompasses changes that come on fairly quickly, either just after the radiation or within a few weeks of conventionally fractionated radiation and resolve within a few months of completing treatment. Nausea, diarrhoea, proctitis, vaginitis and redness or flaking of the skin are all manifestations of the acute radiation reaction. Acute reactions usually settle spontaneously and require supportive symptomatic treatment only, although severe acute reactions can cause ulceration, obstruction, and bleeding. Acute bowel reactions are very common during pelvic radiotherapy. At least 70% of patients have diarrhoea, frequent bowel movements, or colic. The presence of an acute radiation reaction does not necessarily predict that a chronic reaction will occur. The mechanism causing these reactions is different but both reactions relate to the dose received by the tissues.

The chronic radiation reaction may take months or years to develop and includes bowel stricture, bladder stricture, fibrosis and adhesions and various fistulae. The chronic bowel morbidity usually appears within 2 years and the urinary morbidity within 4 years, although both can appear many years later.

Clinical applications of radiotherapy

CERVICAL CANCER

The treatment of cancer of the cervix is very varied between countries, cancer centres and even clinicians. In some situations, particularly for early stage disease, surgery and radiotherapy may be equally effective. The aim is to provide the highest cure rate combined with the lowest associated morbidity (Table 7.1).

Table 7.1   Treatment for cancer of the cervix

Stage	Treatment	Notes
IB	Wertheim's hysterectomy Radical chemoradiotherapy	The results of surgery and radiotherapy are the same but the morbidity is different
IIA:		
Small volume	Either radical surgery or radiotherapy is appropriate	
Bulky	Chemoradiotherapy	
IIB–IIIB	Chemoradiotherapy	
IVA	Exenterative surgery or chemoradiotherapy	
IVB	Palliative therapy	Palliative radiotherapy or chemotherapy

Radiotherapy is the treatment of choice for bulky stage IIA to stage IVA disease. Following surgery with lymph node involvement, high-grade disease or close or involved excision margins, postoperative adjuvant radiotherapy may be offered. Cisplatin chemotherapy is given concurrently with radiotherapy.[2] There is also a role for radiotherapy (and chemoradiotherapy) in patients who develop pelvic recurrence after definitive surgery.

ENDOMETRIAL CANCER

Primary radiotherapy may be used for patients who are unfit for surgery. Although inferior to surgery, it has a 60% 5-year survival for stage I disease. Adjuvant postoperative radiotherapy may be given, with either external beam radiotherapy, vaginal vault brachytherapy or both. Adjuvant radiotherapy is offered to patients with poor prognostic indicators, although there is no international consensus for the indications for adjuvant treatment. Local recurrence was reduced but there was no survival benefit in the UK ASTEC trial or the Canadian Clinical Trials Group EN.5 trial.[3] The PORTEC studies showed a reduction in local recurrence for high-intermediate risk patients from 20% to 5%.[4]

Conventionally, patients are divided into three risk groups for recurrence. The addition of adjuvant therapy is based on those risk categories (Table 7.2).[5]

Most endometrial cancers are well-differentiated endometrioid adenocarcinomas. 15% of endometrial cancers are papillary serous or clear-cell type and considered grade 3. These cancers behave more like ovarian carcinomas than endometrioid endometrial cancers but the value of both adjuvant radiotherapy and chemotherapy in these cancers is uncertain and are best managed in a clinical trial. This subject is explored further in Chapter 10.

Table 7.2	Adjuvant radiotherapy for endometrial cancer		
Risk group	Grade	Stage	Adjuvant radiotherapy
High	3	IC	PORTEC3 trial
	Any grade	≥ IIA	Pelvic radiotherapy
		Lymphovascular space or	Vaginal brachytherapy
		lower segment involvement	Possibly chemotherapy
Intermediate	1–2	IA–B	Vaginal brachytherapy
	3		Possibly pelvic radiotherapy
Low	1–2		No further treatment

VULVAL CANCER

Early stage vulval cancer is treated surgically. Radiotherapy (or chemoradiotherapy) is offered for advanced disease or for those unfit for surgery. Adjuvant postoperative radiotherapy[6] is used for close or positive margins, large deeply invasive lesions with lymphovascular space invasion and in patients with positive inguinal lymph nodes or extracapsular spread from one node. Preoperative chemoradiotherapy for locally advanced carcinoma of the vulva does improve operability[7] but adverse effects are severe. For further details on the role of radiotherapy in vulval cancer management, see Chapter 12.

VAGINAL CANCER

Vaginal cancer is a rare cancer and the evidence base for treatment is thin. Small lesions confined to the vaginal mucosa may be treated with vaginal brachytherapy alone.[8] Chemoradiation is offered for locally advanced vaginal cancer by analogy with carcinoma of the cervix.

OVARIAN CANCER

Radiotherapy was formerly used in the treatment of ovarian cancer. With the onset of effective chemotherapy radiotherapy is only offered palliatively.[9]

RADIOTHERAPY FOR SYMPTOM CONTROL IN A PALLIATIVE CONTEXT

Radiotherapy is widely used in the management of pain from bone metastases. Short courses of radiotherapy may stop patients bleeding from inoperable tumour masses in the vaginal vault. For further details of palliation, see Chapter 14.

References

1. Hall EJ, Giaccia AJ. *Radiobiology for the Radiologist*. 6th edition. Philadelphia, PA: Lippincott Williams and Wilkins; 2006.

2. Green JA, Kirwan JM, Tierney JF, Symonds P, Fresco L, Collingwood M, *et al.* Survival and recurrence after concomitant chemotherapy and radiotherapy for cancer of the uterine cervix: a systematic review and meta-analysis. *Lancet* 2001;358:781–6.

3. ASTEC/EN.5 Study Group, Blake P, Swart AM, Orton J, Kitchener H, Whelan T, Lukka H, *et al.* Adjuvant external beam radiotherapy in the treatment of endometrial cancer (MRC ASTEC and NCIC CTG EN.5 randomised trials): pooled trial results, systematic review, and meta-analysis. *Lancet* 2009;373:137–46.

4. Creutzberg CL, van Putten WL, Koper PC, Lybeert ML, Jobsen JJ, Wárlám-Rodenhuis CC, *et al.* Surgery and postoperative radiotherapy versus surgery alone for patients with stage-1 endometrial carcinoma: multicentre randomised trial. PORTEC Study Group. Post Operative Radiation Therapy in Endometrial Carcinoma. *Lancet* 2000;355:1404–11.

5. Kong A, Powell M, Blake P. The role of postoperative radiotherapy in carcinoma of the endometrium. *Clin Oncol (R Coll Radiol)* 2008;20:457–62.

6. Heaps JM, Fu YS, Montz FJ, Hacker NF, Berek JS. Surgical-pathologic variables predictive of local recurrence in squamous cell carcinoma of the vulva. *Gynecol Oncol* 1990;38:309–14.

7. van Doorn HC, Ansink A, Verhaar-Langereis M, Stalpers L. Neoadjuvant chemoradiation for advanced primary vulval cancer. *Cochrane Database Syst Rev* 2006;(3):CD003752.

8. Frank SJ, Jhingran A, Levenback C, Eifel PJ. Definitive radiation therapy for squamous cell carcinoma of the vagina. *Int J Radiat Oncol Biol Phys* 2005;62:138–47.

9. Tinger A, Waldron T, Peluso N, Katin MJ, Dosoretz DE, Blitzer PH, *et al*. Effective palliative radiation therapy in advanced and recurrent ovarian carcinoma. *Int J Radiat Oncol Biol Phys* 2001;51:1256–63.

8 Chemotherapy: principles and applications

Introduction

Chemotherapy is used in a variety of situations in gynaecological oncology (Box 8.1). The best known is in the treatment of gestational trophoblastic disease, where single-agent treatment is highly successful for low-risk cases and multi-agent regimens are used in the treatment of higher-risk cases. Gestational trophoblastic disease is one of the few solid tumours that is regularly cured by chemotherapy alone. It is, however, an uncommon tumour. The most common use in gynaecology is in the treatment of epithelial and non-epithelial ovarian cancers.

BOX 8.1 USES OF CHEMOTHERAPY IN GYNAECOLOGICAL ONCOLOGY

- Adjuvant and neoadjuvant treatment in ovarian cancer
- Primary treatment of gestational trophoblastic disease
- Relapsed ovarian cancer
- Advanced or relapsed cervical cancer
- Chemoradiation in cervical and vulval cancer
- Advanced and relapsed endometrial cancer
- Sarcomas and non-epithelial ovarian tumours

Chemotherapy is used in an adjuvant setting (after a primary surgical procedure that may or may not have removed all macroscopic disease), in a 'neoadjuvant' fashion (prior to a surgical procedure) and in relapsed or recurrent disease. In cervical cancer, chemotherapy is usually reserved for selected cases of relapsed disease, although, latterly, it has been employed concurrently with radiotherapy in primary treatment (chemoradiation). This principle is also being applied to selected cases of vulval cancer, although less frequently.

In endometrial cancer, chemotherapy is used to treat advanced or relapsed cases where surgery and or radiotherapy are considered inappropriate, although hormone treatment is also used in these situations. Finally, chemotherapy may be used as sole or part therapy for gynaecological sarcomas. It should be stressed that the evidence supporting the use of chemotherapy in advanced endometrial cancers, sarcomas and some non-epithelial tumours is weak. This is largely a result of the infrequency with which these conditions are encountered.

Treatment intent

In some situations, the intent of treatment may be curative, an example being trophoblastic tumours, while in others the intent is palliative, for example in recurrent epithelial ovarian cancer. It is one of the most basic principles of cancer care that this intent should be clearly understood at the outset. This is not only because clear and understandable patient information requires it but also because, without understanding intent, it is impossible to balance risks with benefit. Most, if not all, cytotoxic drugs have adverse effects, some of which can be severe and life threatening. These risks may be acceptable to the woman (and her carers) if the benefit is potential cure; they may not be so if palliation is the primary objective (see Chapter 14).

Toxicity

In all the situations above, conventional chemotherapy used to kill tumour cells will also kill normal, healthy cells. This gives rise to treatment-related toxicity such as myelosuppression, emesis, alopecia and peripheral neuropathy. A balance must be achieved between the effect upon tumour cells and the potential morbidity from treatment-specific toxicities. Some toxic effects of chemotherapy, such as emesis, can be controlled effectively by the use of 5-HT antagonists such as ondansetron, while others, such as severe myelosuppression, can be life threatening. Drugs with differing toxicities are often used in combination to try to maximise the cytotoxic effect upon the tumour without an associated increase in morbidity.

Many features combine to allow the selection of appropriate agents, toxicity being one important parameter. The objective is of course to choose the least toxic regimen (single agent or combined) that has known activity in the disease. The mechanism of action of various drugs differs, as do their pharmacokinetic properties. In most instances when chemotherapy fails, it is because of the development of drug resistance and thus the prevention of resistance is high on the agenda when treatment is being planned. Strategies to try to prevent the development of drug resistance include the use of non-crossreacting agents in multi-drug regimens, drugs with different toxicities, dose, route of administration and

Table 8.1   Complications of chemotherapy

Organ/system	Complication
Haematological	Myelosuppression, common with carboplatin, can cause granulocytopenia Granulocytopenia: predisposes to sepsis. Use prophylactic, broad-spectrum antibiotics in febrile granulocytopenic patients Thrombocytopenia: with a risk of spontaneous haemorrhage Anaemia: usually presents after several courses of chemotherapy
Gastrointestinal	Nausea and vomiting, common adverse effects. 5-HT$_3$ antagonists are effective treatment Mucositis: mouth and pharyngeal ulceration Oesophagitis, causing dysphagia, bowel ulceration resulting in diarrhoea or necrotising enterocolitis (NEC) in severe cases with granulocytopenia. Treatment is with intravenous hydration, electrolyte replacement, antimotility drugs e.g. codeine phosphate and vancomycin in NEC
Hepatotoxicity	Elevation of liver enzymes may occur
Neurotoxicity	Many cytotoxics cause some central or peripheral neurotoxicity Cisplatin produces ototoxicity, peripheral neuropathy, and, rarely, retrobulbar neuritis and blindness Paclitaxel associated with peripheral sensory neuropathy Neurotoxicity increased with combination cisplatin therapy
Immunosuppression	Suppression of cellular and humoral immunity predispose to opportunistic infection
Hypersensitivity reactions	Associated with carboplatin, paclitaxel and anaphylaxis with cisplatin
Alopecia	Usually reversible, common with paclitaxel; associated with significant psychological morbidity
Gonadal dysfunction	Infertility: many cytotoxics cause infertility. Successful pregnancies have been achieved after cisplatin-based chemotherapy Teratogenicity: all cytotoxics carry the risk of teratogenicity
Second malignancies	Cisplatin is associated with the development of acute leukaemia

dose scheduling to maximise the pharmacokinetic properties of the drugs. Despite these efforts, recurrence and relapse are often seen in the treatment of solid tumours, gynaecological cancers included. The complications of chemotherapy are described in Table 8.1.

Epithelial ovarian cancer

See also Chapter 9, Ovarian Cancer Standards of Care.

Almost 75% of women with ovarian cancer have advanced disease at presentation. In this situation, surgery alone is not curative. A large meta-analysis of studies involving almost 7000 women with ovarian cancer found that cytoreductive surgery had only a small effect on the survival of women with advanced ovarian cancer; the type of chemotherapy was found to be more important.[1] Around 70% of women exhibit a response to chemotherapy administered in the adjuvant situation. However, only modest improvements in survival are observed for most women with advanced ovarian cancer and the overall 5-year survival rate has remained poor, at around 25%, for the last 30 years.[2] Chemotherapy in ovarian cancer is platinum-based and, to date, the addition of newer chemotherapeutic agents has resulted in only modest increases in survival.

During the 1980s, cyclophosphamide and cisplatin given in combination became first-line therapy. Cyclophosphamide is an alkylating agent, which acts by cross-linkage of DNA. Cisplatin, developed in the 1960s, has a similar mode of action to the alkylating agents. The adverse effects of cisplatin include nephrotoxicity, emesis, neurotoxicity and ototoxicity (Table 8.1).

Carboplatin is an analogue of cisplatin. It is less nephro- and neurotoxic and causes less vomiting than cisplatin. Following studies showing comparable activity to cisplatin, carboplatin was used in the International Collaboration on Ovarian Neoplasms (ICON 2) trial as a single agent versus a combination of cyclophosphamide, doxorubicin and cisplatin (CAP). There was no difference in outcome between the two groups.[3]

Paclitaxel, one of the taxane group of drugs, was introduced as a first-line therapy in combination with carboplatin. Extracted from the bark of the Western Yew (*Taxus brevifolia*), it acts by stabilising cell microtubules and thus interferes with cell replication. It can cause severe hypersensitivity reactions and its adverse effects include alopecia, neutropenia, myalgia and peripheral neuropathy. The National Institute for Health and Clinical Excellence (NICE) recommends the combination of carboplatin and paclitaxel as first-line adjuvant therapy in epithelial ovarian cancer.

Current research in chemotherapy for advanced ovarian cancer focuses on:

- development of new drugs and combinations of drugs: the combi-nation of carboplatin and paclitaxel with drugs such as gemcitabine, docetaxel and topotecan to form 'triplet' chemotherapy regimens
- neoadjuvant chemotherapy: conventional chemotherapy given in three to four cycles prior to surgical debulking of advanced ovarian cancer, followed by three or four further cycles
- intraperitoneal chemotherapy: conventional drugs administered into the peritoneal cavity following surgery via peritoneal catheters

- gene therapy: novel therapeutic agents developed against tumour vasculature or targeting tumour cells directly are undergoing clinical trials at present.

In the UK and Europe, there is considerable interest in the role of primary (neoadjuvant) chemotherapy and interval debulking surgery. In the UK the CHORUS (Chemotherapy or Upfront Surgery) trial, and the EORTC trial examined the role of neoadjuvant chemotherapy.[4] The EORTC trial shows that disease-free survival and overall survival were similar for both groups (12 and 30 months). Fewer complications were seen in the neoadjuvant group compared with the upfront surgery group, including a significant reduction in postoperative deaths (2.7% versus 6%). The CHORUS study was still open to recruitment at the time of writing but, for many centres in the UK, neoadjuvant chemotherapy is now established as first-line treatment in women with widespread disease on imaging. Interval debulking surgery is considered further in Chapter 9.

EARLY-STAGE OVARIAN CANCER

In contrast to advanced disease, the benefit of adjuvant chemotherapy has been debated in early stage disease. Five-year survival rates of over 90% can be achieved in stage I disease. Presented at the European Cancer Conference in October 2001, the ICON 1 and Adjuvant ChemoTherapy In Ovarian Neoplasm (ACTION) studies helped to clarify the situation.[5] For stage I tumours with certain high-risk features such as clear cell histology, there is a clear survival advantage in those women who received adjuvant chemotherapy.

RECURRENT OVARIAN CANCER

In recurrent disease, chemotherapy for ovarian cancer is always palliative. Platinum-based chemotherapy may be given as a second-line treatment. Response rates are closely related to the time from primary treatment to relapse. Response rates vary from 25% (in those relapsing within one year) to 60% for those with a disease-free interval of more than two years.[6] For platinum-resistant disease, oral etoposide shows response rates of around 27% and is currently used following failure of first- or second-line platinum-based regimens.[7]

Tamoxifen 40 mg daily may have some benefit in women who are considered unfit for further chemotherapy, as a palliative treatment.[8]

Cervical cancer

In general terms, until recently, the first-line therapy for cervical cancer was a choice between surgery and radiotherapy for early-stage disease with radiotherapy for advanced disease. Chemotherapy was used mainly as an adjuvant treatment in certain high-risk situations or in the context of recurrent disease. Chemotherapy with combinations such as bleomycin [B], ifosfamide [I] and cisplatin [P] (BIP regimen) was used. In addition to the nephrotoxicity of cisplatin, bleomycin can cause pulmonary morbidity, while ifosfamide can cause neurological morbidity.

In an almost unprecedented action, the *New England Journal of Medicine* published on the internet the results of three studies on chemoradiation in cervical cancer in advance of their publication in the journal itself.[9–11] Following this, the National Cancer Institute of the National Institutes for Health in Washington, USA, issued a clinical announcement stating that 'strong consideration' should be given to the incorporation of concurrent cisplatin-based chemotherapy with radiation therapy in women who require radiation therapy for treatment of cervical cancer.

Taken together, the results of five trials involving almost 2000 women with stage I–IV cervical cancer show a 30–50% reduction in the relative risks of relapse or death. These results do, however, appear to come at the price of increased morbidity, such as bowel toxicity, which may require bowel resection and has in some cases resulted in death. The balance between the improved outcome versus increased morbidity is the subject of debate in the UK, although many gynaecological oncology centres have included chemoradiation in their treatment protocols for the management of cervical cancer.

For women with recurrent cervical cancer, or stage IVB disease at presentation, there has been interest in using topotecan. The position in England regarding the use of topotecan in this situation has been clarified following publication of a NICE guideline on the subject.[12] NICE has recommended that topotecan, in combination with cisplatin, be considered as a treatment option for women with recurrent or stage IVB cervical cancer but only if they have not previously received cisplatin.

Endometrial cancer

Unlike women with epithelial ovarian cancer, the majority of those with endometrial cancer present with early-stage disease. Treatment for this group is surgical, with total abdominal hysterectomy, bilateral salpingo-oophorectomy, peritoneal washings and pelvic lymphadenectomy forming part of the staging procedure.

Currently, prognostic factors such as tumour grade, depth of myometrial invasion, lymph node involvement and peritoneal cytology are used to determine the need for adjuvant therapy. This takes the form of radiotherapy, either to the vaginal vault or pelvis. There is no evidence that such treatment prolongs survival.

Several chemotherapeutic approaches have been investigated in endometrial cancer in attempts to improve survival. Drugs used include cisplatin, carboplatin, doxorubicin and paclitaxel. Progestogen therapy using drugs such as medroxyprogesterone acetate (MPA) and megestrol have shown response rates of up to 30% but without evidence of increased survival.

Both platinum- and paclitaxel-based drug combinations have shown similar response rates but, again, these have not translated into improved survival.[13,14]

Vulval cancer

Where possible, the management of vulval cancer is usually surgical in the first instance, with adjuvant radiotherapy in situations where the excision margin is incomplete/inadequate on the vulva and/or the inguinal/pelvic lymph nodes are involved (see Chapter 12).

Chemotherapy, using 5-fluorouracil, cisplatin or both, in combination with radiotherapy, has been used in women who are unfit for surgery or in those in whom exenterative surgery would have to be performed to excise all tumour. Using this approach, response rates of 50–90% have been reported. In cases where complete response has been achieved, some authors suggest that surgical excision of the primary tumour site is not necessary.[15]

This approach has led to interest in preoperative treatment for women with extensive tumours in whom radical primary surgery would be required to remove all tumour. By giving chemoradiation preoperatively, several studies have shown that the need for radical surgery decreases; for example, leading to preservation of the anal sphincter and avoiding the necessity for major plastic reconstructive procedures.[16]

Rare tumours

GESTATIONAL TROPHOBLASTIC TUMOURS

Gestational trophoblastic tumours are the malignant gestational trophoblastic diseases, complete and partial hydatidiform mole being preinvasive. Comprising invasive mole, choriocarcinoma and placental site trophoblastic tumours, these tumours are important, since the vast majority of women with these conditions are curable with chemotherapy. Women in the UK are referred for follow-up to centres in Dundee, Sheffield or London.

Certain indications for chemotherapy have been established. These include:

- choriocarcinoma on histology
- serum β-human chorionic gonadotrophin (hCG) greater than 20 000 iu/l more than 4 weeks after evacuation of the uterus

- metastatic disease
- persistent haemorrhage
- static/rising β-hCG following evacuation of the uterus.

If any of these indications exist, then women are given chemotherapy based upon their level of risk. The risk category is calculated using a scoring system that takes many factors into account, including the woman's age, the β-hCG level and whether the preceding pregnancy had been molar.

Women judged to be at 'low-risk' are treated with intramuscular methotrexate with folinic acid rescue.[17] The 'high-risk' group of women, together with the small number who develop resistance to methotrexate, are treated with an alternating regimen of etoposide [E], methotrexate [M] and actinomycin D [A] and cyclophosphamide [C] and vincristine [O]. The EMA-CO regimen can also be augmented with intrathecal methotrexate in women with cerebral metastases.[18]

NON-EPITHELIAL OVARIAN TUMOURS

The malignant non-epithelial tumours comprise mainly sex-cord stromal and germ-cell tumours. They generally occur in younger women and, although not common, they form an important group of ovarian tumours because, unlike the epithelial ovarian tumours, long-term survival and cure can often be achieved.

Of the sex-cord stromal tumours, granulosa cell tumours may require chemotherapy. Combination therapy with bleomycin [B], etoposide [E] and cisplatin [P] (BEP regimen) is active in this situation.[19]

The malignant germ-cell tumours include dysgerminomas and a group of non-dysgerminomas which includes endodermal sinus tumours and teratomas. Combination chemotherapy with BEP or cisplatin [P], vinblastine [V] and bleomycin [B] (PVB regimen) allow response rates of around 90% to be achieved.[20,21] It is worth restating the recommendation that, in young women of childbearing age, the initial laparotomy for an ovarian tumour should consider fertility preservation, owing to the potentially curable nature of some of the non-epithelial ovarian tumours.

KEY POINTS

Ovarian cancer

- Adjuvant therapy recommended for high-risk early stage ovarian cancer.
- For advanced disease, poor 5-year survival of around 25%.
- Current adjuvant chemotherapy in advanced disease – carboplatin and paclitaxel.
- Response rates in relapsed disease relate to time since last chemotherapy.
- Neoadjuvant surgery in advanced disease is associated with lower morbidity than upfront surgery.

Cervical cancer

- Concurrent cisplatin-based chemotherapy should be considered in all women who require adjuvant radiotherapy.
- Treatment-related morbidity is likely to be higher in this group.
- Topotecan may be considered for women with recurrent or stage IVB disease in combination with cisplatin (if they have not received cisplatin previously).

Endometrial cancer

- Progestogen and platinum-based therapies show response rates of up to 30%.
- No evidence that this translates into prolonged survival.

Vulval cancer

- Good responses to 5-fluorouracil-based chemoradiation regimens.
- Preservation of function and avoidance of extended radical procedures possible using chemoradiation.

Gestational trophoblastic tumours

- Follow-up and treatment via centres in Dundee, Sheffield and London.
- Several indications for chemotherapy.
- If indicated, chemotherapy based on low- or high-risk scores.
- High cure rates.

Non-epithelial ovarian tumours

- Chemosensitive tumours often associated with high cure rates.
- Always consider fertility-preserving surgery in women of childbearing age.

References

1. Hunter RW, Alexander ND, Soutter WP. Meta-analysis of surgery in advanced ovarian carcinoma: is maximum cytoreductive surgery an independent determinant of prognosis? *Am J Obstet Gynecol* 1992;166:504–11.

2. Thomas H. Cancer of the ovary: advances in chemotherapy. *Trends in Urology, Gynaecology and Sexual Health* 1998;3:11–16.

3. International Collaborative Ovarian Neoplasm Study Collaborators. ICON 2: randomised trial of single-agent carboplatin against three-drug combination of CAP (cyclophosphamide, doxorubicin, and cisplatin) in women with ovarian cancer. *Lancet* 1998;352:1571–6.

4. Vergote I, Trope CG, Amant GB, Kristensen JE, Sardi T, Ehlen N, *et al.* EORTC_GCG/NCIC-CTG randomized trial comparing primary debulking surgery with neoadjuvant chemotherapy in stage IIIC-IV ovarian, fallopian tube, and peritoneal cancer (OVCA). Proceedings of the 12th Biennial Meeting of the International Gynecologic Cancer Society, Bangkok 2008. Abstract No. 1767 [www.igcs.org/Abstract/meeting_2008_1767.html].

5. Colombo N. Randomised trial of paclitaxel (PTX) and carboplatin (CBDCA) vs a control arm of carboplatin or CAP (cyclophosphamide, doxorubicin, and cisplatin):the third International Collaborative Ovarian Neoplasm Study (ICON 3). *Proc Am Soc Clin Oncol* 2000;19:379a.

6. Blackledge G, Lawton F, Redman C, Kelly K. Responses of patients in phase II studies of chemotherapy in ovarian cancer: implications for patient treatment and the design of phase II trials. *Br J Cancer* 1989;59:650–3.

7. Rose P, Blessing J, Mayer A, Homesley H. Prolonged oral etoposide as secondline therapy in platinum-resistant or platinum-sensitive ovarian carcinoma: a Gynecologic Oncology Group Study. *J Clin Oncol* 1998;16:405–10.

8. Markman M, Iseminger KA, Hatch KD, Creasman WT, Barnes W, Dubeshter B. Tamoxifen in platinum-refractory ovarian cancer: a Gynecologic Oncology Group Ancillary Report. *Gynecol Oncol* 1996;62:4–6.

9. Rose PG, Bundy BN, Watkins EB, Thigpen JT, Deppe G, Maiman MA, *et al.* Concurrent cisplatin-based radiotherapy and chemotherapy for locally advanced cervical cancer. *N Engl J Med* 1999;340:1144–53.

10. Keys HM, Bundy BN, Stehman FB, Muderspach LI, Chafe WE, Suggs CL 3rd, *et al.* Cisplatin, radiation and adjuvant hysterectomy compared with radiotherapy and adjuvant hysterectomy for bulky stage 1b cervical cancer. *N Engl J Med* 1999;340:1154–61.

11. Morris M, Eifel PJ, Lu J, Grigsby PW, Levenback C, Stevens RE, *et al.* Pelvic radiation with concurrent chemotherapy compared with pelvic and para-aortic radiation for high-risk cervical cancer. *N Engl J Med* 1999;340:1137–43.

12. National Institute for Health and Clinical Excellence. *Topotecan for the Treatment of Recurrent and Stage IVB Cervical Cancer*. NICE Technology Appraisal Guidance 183. London: NICE; 2009 [http://guidance.nice.org.uk/TA183].

13. Burke TW, Munkarah A, Kavanagh JJ, Morris M, Levenback C, Tornos C, *et al.* Treatment of advanced or recurrent endometrial cancer with single agent carboplatin. *Gynecol Oncol* 1993;51:397–400.

14. Ball HG, Blessing JA, Lentz SS, Mutch DG. A phase II trial of paclitaxel in patients with advanced or recurrent adenocarcinoma of the endometrium: a Gynecologic Oncology Group study. *Gynecol Oncol* 1996;62:278–81.

15. Cunningham MJ, Goyer RP, Gibbons SK, Kredentser DC, Malfetano JH, Keys H. Primary radiation, cisplatin, and 5-fluorouracil for advanced squamous carcinoma of the vulva. *Gynecol Oncol* 1997;66:258–61.

16. Montana GS, Thomas GM, Moore DH, Saxer A, Mangan CE, Lentz SS, *et al.* Preoperative chemo-radiation for carcinoma of the vulva with N2/N3 nodes: a Gynecologic Oncology Group study. *Int J Radiat Oncol Biol Phys* 2000;48:1007–13.

17. Howie PW. Trophoblastic disease. In: Whitfield CR, editor. *Dewhurst's Textbook of Obstetrics and Gynaecology for Postgraduates*. 5th ed. London: Blackwell; 1995. p. 556–67.

18. Bower M, Newlands ES, Holden L, Short D, Brock C, Rustin GJ, *et al.* EMA/CO for high-risk gestational trophoblastic tumours: results from a cohort of 272 patients. *J Clin Oncol* 1997;15:2636–43.

19. Homesley HD, Bundy BN, Hurteau JA, Roth LM. Bleomycin, etoposide, and cisplatin combination chemotherapy of ovarian granulosa cell tumours and other stromal malignancies: a Gynecologic Oncology Group study. *Gynecol Oncol* 1999;72:131–7.

20. Brewer M, Gershenson DM, Herzog CE, Mitchell MF, Silva EG, Wharton JT. Outcome and reproductive function after chemotherapy for ovarian dysgerminoma. *J Clin Oncol* 1999;17:2670–75.

21. Mayordomo JI, Paz-Ares L, Rivera F, Lopez-Brea M, Lopez Martin E, Mendiola C, *et al.* Ovarian and extragonadal malignant germ-cell tumors in females: a single-institution experience with 43 patients. *Ann Oncol* 1994;5:225–31.

9 Ovarian cancer standards of care

Introduction

Ovarian cancer is the fourth most common cause of cancer deaths in women and the leading cause of gynaecological cancer death in Europe,[1,2] with a lifetime prevalence in the developed world of 1–2%.[3] The incidence increases with age, peaking in the eighth decade, with a median age at diagnosis of 63 years. It is often described as a silent killer but early symptoms of abdominal bloating, urinary frequency, a sensation of fullness and pelvic or abdominal pain are frequently reported.[4] As these symptoms are non-specific, they are often dismissed by both women and healthcare professionals. When ovarian cancer is detected, it is usually at an advanced stage with a poor prognosis. In the UK, ovarian cancer kills 4400 women each year,[5] more women than all of the other gynaecological malignancies combined.

Survival for ovarian cancer patients in the UK has increased over time but the average survival still lags behind the Nordic countries[1] and the USA. Childbearing, breastfeeding and use of the oral contraceptive pill all protect against the development of ovarian cancer. This is thought to be due to a reduced number of ovulatory cycles minimising the damage and repair cycle of the ovarian epithelium. It is likely, therefore, that the increased incidence of ovarian cancer over the past few decades is partly due to reduced parity. Patients with ovarian cancer are best cared for by multidisciplinary teams.

Over the past 30 years, the role of surgical debulking has been established. Following the introduction of more effective chemotherapy, the timing of surgery and chemotherapy has been questioned. Primary debulking, where feasible, remains the standard treatment. Where this is not possible, interval debulking has been defined as a further attempt following chemotherapy, while neoadjuvant chemotherapy followed by surgery (NACT-S) is the term applied to the strategy of primary chemotherapy in potentially resectable cases. Radiotherapy has a more limited role primarily in palliation of advanced disease.

Classification of ovarian cancer

Primary ovarian tumours are a heterogeneous group which includes epithelial tumours, sex-cord stromal and germ-cell tumours. Tumours not specific to the ovaries also occur, such as sarcomas and lymphomas. Metastatic tumours from breast, stomach and endometrial primaries are not uncommon.

EPITHELIAL TUMOURS

The majority of ovarian tumours (59% of all ovarian tumours and up to 90% of all primary ovarian malignancies) are epithelial. These arise from the cells covering the surface of the ovary and probably also from the fimbrial end of the fallopian tube and less frequently from endometriotic implants within the ovaries. Pathological diagnosis should be made according to the World Health Organization classification. Epithelial tumours can be further classified as:

- serous
- mucinous
- endometrioid
- clear cell
- transitional cell (Brenner)
- mixed
- undifferentiated carcinomas.

Serous tumours are the most common subtype and account for about 50%.

GRADE

Malignant tumours are characterised by their grade: this describes the microscopic pattern of growth (architecture) and cellular features (cytology) and varies from well differentiated (grade G1) to moderately and poorly differentiated (G2 and G3 respectively). Well-differentiated tumours have a better prognosis than G2 or G3 tumours.

DISSEMINATION OF THE DISEASE

Epithelial ovarian cancer spreads:

- directly to the uterus and fallopian tubes
- via the peritoneum to the rest of the peritoneal cavity, especially the omentum
- via the lymphatics to pelvic and para-aortic lymph nodes
- by haematogenous spread to the liver, lungs and other organs.

PRIMARY PERITONEAL TUMOURS

Primary peritoneal cancer can be clinically and histologically indistinguishable from metastatic epithelial ovarian cancer. It is diagnosed when a condition identical to disseminated peritoneal ovarian cancer arises in the absence of any clear ovarian primary. The treatment is the same as for ovarian cancer, although, as there is often no mass to debulk, chemotherapy is more often used as the primary treatment.

BORDERLINE TUMOURS

Borderline ovarian tumours also arise from the ovarian epithelium and are a subcategory that may be separated from clearly benign and clearly malignant tumours. The behaviour of these tumours is more indolent but they may nevertheless be associated with extra-ovarian disease of similar histology, with implants in the omentum and peritoneum. Thus, it is possible to have advanced-stage borderline disease. This terminology has led to much confusion regarding the natural history of the category. Other terms such as 'carcinoma of low malignant potential' or 'atypical proliferating tumour' have been suggested and these may be easier to conceptualise. However, the term 'borderline' is accepted by the World Health Organization and will remain for the foreseeable future.

Borderline tumours are typically found in a younger population than frank epithelial cancers, with one-third occurring in women under the age of 40 years. It is probable that they represent a form of premalignant disease for low-grade ovarian carcinomas. The overall prognosis is good but recurrences have been reported as late as 30 years after initial presentation. A woman with a borderline tumour diagnosed after a unilateral salpingo-oophorectomy may be advised that the recurrence risk without further surgery is approximately 7%.

There is no evidence that treatment of borderline tumours with adjuvant chemotherapy is beneficial. A particular challenge is posed by the group of women who have serous borderline tumours which exhibit invasive omental or peritoneal implants. In a study of 44 women with serous borderline tumours, four women with invasive implants died of their disease between 3 and 9 years later, despite chemotherapy.[6]

NON-EPITHELIAL OVARIAN NEOPLASMS

The relative rarity of this group of cancers results in a relative paucity of data upon which to determine management. The above recommendations about adequate surgery and debulking still apply. The relatively early age of presentation of germ-cell tumours necessitates conservative surgery in the majority of patients. Young women who present with solid or semi-solid tumours should have other tumour markers measured.

SEX-CORD STROMAL TUMOURS

Sex-cord stromal tumours account for approximately 7% of all malignant ovarian tumours. They arise from a combination of the hormone-producing cells of the ovary and stromal fibroblasts. Around 70% of all malignant sex-cord stromal tumours are granulosa cell tumours. Most occur in women in their sixth decade, although a small proportion arises in young women and prepubertal girls. Granulosa-cell tumours are frequently estrogen secreting, although androgen-secreting varieties do occur. High levels of estrogen can lead to endometrial pathology, including endometrial hyperplasia and carcinoma. Common presenting symptoms include abdominal distension, acute abdominal pain and abnormal vaginal bleeding. Most present at an early stage and have an excellent prognosis. Treatment is principally surgical with platinum-based chemotherapy for advanced or recurrent disease.[7] Surgical treatment is as for epithelial ovarian cancer, although, in young women with early disease, fertility preservation is an option. Other stromal tumours are rare and include thecomas, fibromas, Sertoli–Leydig cell tumours and gynandroblastomas.

MALIGNANT GERM-CELL TUMOURS

Malignant germ-cell tumours occur chiefly in girls and young women. The most common variety is the dysgerminoma, the counterpart to the seminoma in the male. Other types include the yolk sac tumour, embryonal carcinoma, polyembryoma, non-gestational choriocarcinoma and teratoma. They usually present with abdominal pain, which is sometimes acute, and a palpable pelvic mass. Several of these tumours secrete tumour markers, which are useful in diagnosis and monitoring (such as alphafetoprotein, human chorionic gonadotrophin and lactic dehydrogenase). Treatment is primarily surgical. As over 60% are confined to one ovary at diagnosis, fertility-sparing surgery is usual, with unilateral salpingo-oophorectomy or even ovarian cystectomy in selected cases with otherwise normal ovaries. Dysgerminomas are unusual ovarian tumours in that they are highly radiosensitive. However, as this usually results in premature ovarian failure, platinum-based chemotherapy is currently the preferred option. Non-dysgerminoma tumours are treated with the chemotherapy combination of bleomycin, etoposide and cisplatin. Response rates are excellent, with cure rates approaching 100% in early stage disease and up to 75% in advanced disease.[8]

Prognostic factors

Many attempts have been made to classify ovarian tumours, usually with the aim of determining prognosis more accurately. Established favourable prognostic factors include:

- surgical stage (FIGO I–IV)
- small tumour volume, both before and after surgery
- younger age
- good performance status (American Society of Anesthesiologists grade)
- cell type other than mucinous or clear cell
- well-differentiated tumours (G1)
- absence of ascites.

Favourable factors for stage I tumours include:

- cell type other than clear cell
- absence of ascites
- low grade
- absence of dense adhesions
- FIGO stage subgroups a or b, rather than c.

Presentation and diagnosis

Since early diagnosis is associated with a better outcome, significant improvements in the cure rate for ovarian cancer are likely to result from prompt diagnosis and referral to suitable specialists. Unfortunately, the symptoms of ovarian cancer are often non-specific and may mimic other conditions (bloating, abdominal pain, change in bowel habit, backache, weight loss and menstrual disorders).[9] An average general practitioner will see a new case of ovarian cancer every 5 years. Thus, the non-specific nature of the symptoms may lead to a delay in diagnosis of up to 1 year.[4] A study by Goff *et al.*[10] suggested that a distinct set of symptoms is experienced, even by women with very early disease. Importantly, symptoms are not usually gynaecological in nature but are often indicative of conditions affecting the abdomen or gastrointestinal tract:

- increased abdominal size or persistent distension
- persistent abdominal and/or pelvic pain
- difficulty eating or feeling full quickly.

Critically, it is not just the presence of symptoms but also their frequency and persistency that is highly indicative of ovarian cancer. The Department of Health is advising women experiencing these symptoms to seek medical advice, particularly if they are experiencing symptoms on most days. In addition, urinary symptoms, changes in bowel habit, extreme fatigue or weight loss are also cited as symptoms that can be indicative of ovarian cancer.

INITIAL ASSESSMENT

It is estimated that 5–10% of women will undergo a surgical procedure for a suspected ovarian neoplasm during their lifetime and 13–21% of these women will be found to have an ovarian malignancy. Since the majority of masses are benign, it is important to try to determine preoperatively whether a woman is at high risk of ovarian malignancy, to ensure proper management.

Routine assessment for women with a pelvic mass should comprise a full history and examination, including vaginal with or without rectal examination. Investigation should include an ultrasound examination of the abdomen and pelvis and serum CA125 levels. Serum CA125 and transvaginal ultrasound remain at the core of all new screening and diagnostic strategies for ovarian cancer. Since 1999, several new markers have been discovered. None has, however, been validated in a prospective randomised screening trial. The ultrasound findings and serum CA125 level together are therefore used to calculate the risk of malignancy index (RMI) taking into account the woman's menopausal status (Figure 9.1).[11]

A score of 200 or greater gives a sensitivity of 85% and a specificity of 97% for ovarian cancer. Using this level as a cut off point, clinicians outside the gynaecology oncology centre who perform surgery for low-risk pelvic masses will use the RMI calculation to determine whether referral to a cancer centre is appropriate. Women with pelvic masses considered likely to be malignant as a result of clinical and ultrasound findings should be referred immediately to the specialist team at the cancer centre, unless the

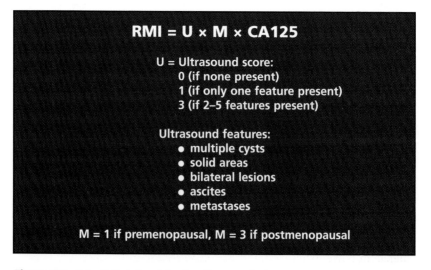

Figure 9.1 Calculating the risk of malignancy index

cause is thought likely to be tumours metastatic to the ovary from non-gynaecological sites. In such cases, combined management with the local cancer team at the referring unit is usually preferable.

Patients who fall into one or other of the above groups should nonetheless not be referred centrally if they are known or suspected to have conditions likely to cause false positive serum CA125 levels. These include endometriosis, adenomyosis, benign ovarian cysts, Meigs syndrome, ovarian hyperstimulation syndrome, fibroids, tubo-ovarian abscess, pancreatitis, chronic liver disease, colitis, diverticulitis, renal disease, systemic autoimmune conditions and malignancies of lung, breast and gastrointestinal tract.

If the woman is admitted as an emergency and the clinical situation permits, the condition should be stabilised and the patient transferred to the care of the gynaecological oncologist.

IF MALIGNANCY IS SUSPECTED

The initial assessment should record:

- relevant present and past medical history
- vaginal and rectal examination
- performance status (American Society of Anesthesiologists grade)
- family history, including first-degree relatives with ovarian, breast or colon cancer.

Before surgery or chemotherapy, the following should be arranged:

- complete full blood count (FBC) and differential
- biochemistry for hepatic (liver function tests) and renal function (urea and electrolytes)
- serum CA125
- if the woman is less than 40 years of age with a partly or wholly solid tumour, add alphafetoprotein, human chorionic gonadotrophin, lactate dehydrogenase (LDH)
- if there is a possibility of primary bowel pathology, add carcinoembryonic antigen (CEA)
- if there is a possibility of disseminated upper gastrointestinal malignancy, add CA19.9
- chest X-ray
- computed tomography (CT) of the abdomen and pelvis.

If ascites or pleural effusions are present then consider paracentesis or pleural tap for cytology and symptomatic relief. Breast, bronchus, stomach and large bowel cancers often spread to the ovaries. If there has been a suspicious change in bowel habit (or low CA125:CEA ratio) other imaging modalities may be appropriate. A ratio of CA125:CEA of greater than 25 favours the diagnosis of ovarian cancer. Barium studies or endoscopy should be performed in those suspected of having a primary gastrointestinal malignancy.

If not performed before surgery, all patients should have a CT scan of the abdomen and pelvis before chemotherapy. The routine use of positron emission tomography for initial staging is not recommended.

There are some patients who may benefit from immediate primary or neoadjuvant chemotherapy and deferred surgery. These patients include the medically unfit and women with disseminated multifocal small volume disease, usually associated with massive ascites. Image-controlled, directed laparoscopic biopsies may be appropriate to obtain a histological diagnosis. However, it needs to be stressed that cyst aspiration is not routinely recommended when ovarian cancer is suspected. Negative cytology does not safely exclude the diagnosis and cyst leakage may disseminate and upstage the cancer.

Referral to the multidisciplinary team

A multidisciplinary team meeting at the outset of treatment is beneficial for strategic planning of the clinical management. The team usually includes nurse specialists, medical oncologists, histopathologists, radiologists, palliative care specialists and gynaecological oncologists in collaboration with the patients and their families. Case discussion for new patients should include review of:

- imaging (CT and ultrasound)
- cytology from ascites or pleural fluid
- histology from biopsy
- management options (upfront surgery or chemotherapy)
- suitability for recruitment into clinical trials
- disease recurrence.

All women should be offered the support of, and have access to, a clinical nurse specialist for psychological support and to help facilitate their cancer journey, especially as many women may experience co-morbid psychological disorders such as anxiety and depression.[12]

Surgery for ovarian carcinoma

There are a number of indications for surgery:

- establishment of the diagnosis
- accurate staging
- primary cytoreduction
- interval and secondary cytoreduction
- palliative and salvage surgery.

DIAGNOSIS

Whether performing surgery to investigate an adnexal mass or the origin of a widespread carcinoma with ascites, exploratory surgery with tissue biopsy and subsequent expert histopathological examination is crucial to making a diagnosis in most cases.

STAGING

Accurate staging procedures are important in determining the future management of any ovarian carcinoma.[13] The incision used should be of a suitable type (vertical) and size to allow adequate exploration of the entire abdominal cavity and removal of ovarian masses intact where possible (Figures 9.2 and 9.3). A sample of any ascites present should be sent for cytological analysis and, in the absence of ascites, peritoneal washings are performed. The abdominal contents, peritoneal surfaces and retro-peritoneal spaces should then be carefully and systematically examined to determine the extent of any macroscopic disease. Infracolic omentectomy is routinely indicated for staging unless there is inoperable carcinomatosis. Sampling of the pelvic and para-aortic nodes may be required.

Surgery should be performed by an appropriately trained gynaecological oncologist with experience in the management of ovarian cancer. Staging is described using the FIGO classification (Table 9.1).

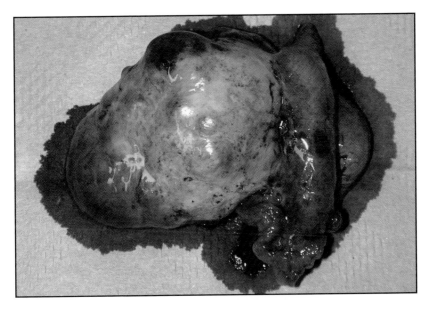

Figure 9.2 Intact malignant ovarian cyst stage I

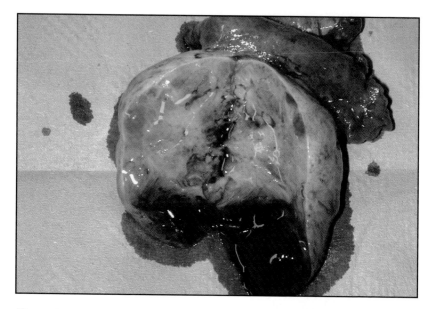

Figure 9.3 Same cyst shown in Figure 9.2 opened showing solid components

PRIMARY CYTOREDUCTION

Standard primary surgery should involve total abdominal hysterectomy, bilateral salpingo-oophorectomy, infracolic omentectomy and tumour debulking. Surgical staging is also mandatory and includes cytology washings in apparent early stage disease, and retroperitoneal node assessment.

OPTIMAL DEBULKING

The standard form of surgical intervention in advanced ovarian cancer is to undertake a pelvic clearance and remove all visible tumour. When the latter is not feasible, then a 'debulking operation' is performed (Figure 9.4). This is a procedure whereby the intra-abdominal tumour load is reduced to what is termed 'optimum residual disease'. 'Optimal debulking' has been defined in different ways at different times in the literature, but currently is generally understood to mean cytoreduction to tumour deposits 1 cm or less.

Compared with other intra-abdominal solid tumours, this aggressive surgical approach is unique to ovarian cancer. Many retrospective studies[15] and meta-analyses may indicate that patients with 'optimum' debulking survive longer than those with a greater amount of residual disease. For instance, the widely quoted meta-analysis of nearly 7000 stage III/IV ovarian cancer patients demonstrated that each 10% improvement in the total debulking rate was associated with a 5.5% improvement in median

Table 9.1	FIGO staging of ovarian cancer[14]
Stage	Description
I	Confined to the ovaries
IA	One ovary, no ascites present containing malignant cells, no tumour on external surface, capsule intact
IB	Both ovaries, no ascites present containing malignant cells, no tumour on external surfaces, capsule intact
IC	Tumour limited to one or both ovaries with any of the following; tumour on the surface on one or both ovaries, capsule ruptured, ascites present with malignant cells or positive peritoneal washings
II	Growth involving one or both ovaries with pelvic extension
IIA	Extension and/or metastases to uterus and/or fallopian tubes
IIB	Extension to other pelvic tissues
IIC	Tumour stage IIa or IIb but with tumour on surface of one or both ovaries, capsule ruptured, ascites present containing malignant cells or positive peritoneal washings
III	Tumour involving one or both ovaries with microscopically confirmed peritoneal implants outside the pelvis and/or regional lymph node metastasis
IIIA	Microscopic peritoneal metastasis beyond the pelvis
IIIB	Macroscopic peritoneal metastasis beyond the pelvis, 2 cm or less in greatest dimension
IIIC	Abdominal implants greater than 2 cm in diameter and/or regional lymph nodes metastasis
IV	Distant metastasis beyond the peritoneal cavity. Includes liver parenchymal metastasis and/or pleural effusion with positive cytology

survival.[16] The reality, however, is that this surgical intervention has never been tested in a randomised controlled trial. Therefore, rather than 'optimum debulking' enhancing survival, it could be that the ability to achieve this is only reflecting the inherent tumour biology or a more chemosensitive disease. This debate will continue until such studies are completed; however, there is no doubt that surgery plays a central role in the management of ovarian carcinoma.

ULTRARADICAL SURGERY

There is an increasing body of evidence to indicate that while operative management for advanced stage disease is capable of contributing to an improved outcome, it only does so when all macroscopic disease is

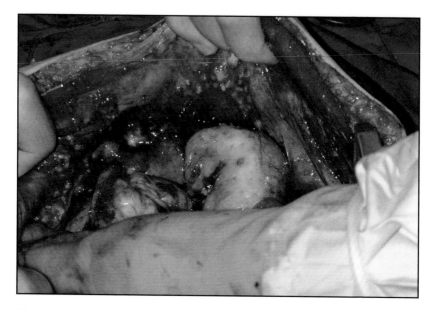

Figure 9.4 Advanced ovarian tumour with seedlings

completely removed.[17] This should be readily achievable in 22–25% of cases of advanced stage III disease.[18] The Gynecologic Oncology Group (GOG) published the largest series to date using six control arms of different prospective randomised trials all using cisplatin and paclitaxel chemotherapy. There were 1895 women with stage III ovarian cancer, of which 23% were cytoreduced to no visible disease. Progression-free survival was 33.0 months, 16.8 months, 14.1 months, and the overall survival was 71.9 months, 42.4 months, 35.0 months for those with no macroscopic disease, 0.1–1.0 cm residual disease and greater than 1 cm residual disease respectively.[17]

The issue of surgery in women with stage IV has shown similar trends but with lower cytoreduction rates. Winter *et al.*[19] reported on 360 patients in the control arms of four GOG studies, again involving intravenous cisplatin and paclitaxel. The maximal cytoreduction rate was only 8%. Once again, the maximum benefit was seen in those patients cytoreduced to no residual disease (progression-free survival 20.1 months and overall survival 64.1 months). Interestingly, there was no difference in survival for patients with 0.1–1.0 cm residual disease compared with 1–5 cm residual disease.

Only two groups have published large series with an initial surgical cytoreduction rate in excess of 80%.[20–22] This involves an ultraradical approach with more aggressive upper abdominal surgery, including splenectomy, cholecystectomy, partial pancreatectomy, radical stripping of the peritoneum (including the diaphragm and multiple bowel resections). This was at the expense of increasing postoperative morbidity and mortality and longer operating time. Their median survival however for stage IIIc disease was 75.8 months.[20]

A consensus is developing in the UK regarding the desirability of pursuing this style of management.

Lymphadenectomy

The question of systematic lymphadenectomy has been examined in a pivotal randomised controlled trial involving 13 centres over 12 years, with 427 patients and a long median (68.4 months) follow-up.[23] There was no overall survival advantage. A modest improvement in progression-free survival in the lymphadenectomy arm was offset by increased morbidity.

Retroperitoneal palpation of node chains should always be carried out but removal of lymph nodes is only indicated where this would potentially affect the stage of disease or result in the removal of bulky disease. Selective removal should not otherwise be justified unless undertaken as part of a research protocol.

CURRENT STANDARD

Systematic lymphadenectomy is not indicated as part of first-line management of ovarian cancer.

Early stage disease, FIGO stage I and IIa epithelial ovarian cancer

Fewer than 30% of women present with stage I or II ovarian cancer.[24] Stage I epithelial ovarian cancer is, however, relatively more frequent in women below the age of 40 years who may wish to retain fertility. Standard management should involve total abdominal hysterectomy, bilateral salpingo-oophorectomy, omentectomy and assessment of the retroperitoneal nodes as described above. In younger women with localised unilateral tumours (FIGO stage I) it is usual to simply remove the affected ovary and to carry out a thorough surgical staging. Wedge biopsy of the contralateral ovary should be performed, if the contralateral ovary is not normal on inspection. When the ovarian tumour is densely adherent to other abdominal or pelvic structures, the patient should be 'upstaged' and treated as a FIGO stage II tumour as the relapse rate seems to be similar.

On the basis of the available evidence, when a woman wishes to retain her fertility, removal of a single abnormal ovary with careful examination of the entire abdominal cavity may not be associated with a high risk of recurrence. Washings and omental biopsy are required for stage confirmation.

As the majority of ovarian cysts will be eventually found to be benign and bearing in mind that up to 50% of stage I ovarian cancer will have a normal serum CA125 level, there is no evidence to justify routine lymphadenectomy, although some clinicians would choose to perform pelvic/para-aortic node sampling in these circumstances. It has, however, become clear that the performance of lymphadenectomy in these patients will result in stage migration whereby more patients will be allocated to stage III disease when lymph node metastasis is discovered. This will apparently improve the survival of all stage groups without altering the overall survival of the whole group.

Stage IV disease

The GOG study on stage IV ovarian cancer found that the small number of women (6%) who could be completely debulked had a survival advantage.[19] There was little advantage for those women with any residual disease remaining. However, in young women with stage IV disease (cytology positive pleural effusion), no organ dysfunction, small volume disease and good performance status surgical debulking should be considered in the same way as FIGO stage III disease. The other alternative would be NACT-S if a response was obtained with chemotherapy.

CURRENT STANDARD

Young women with good performance status and pleural effusion as the only site of disease outside the abdomen should be considered for debulking surgery.

Second-look laparotomy or laparoscopy

Second-look laparotomy or laparoscopy describes an operation taking place after the completion of first-line chemotherapy, the aims of which are to assess disease status (response to chemotherapy). On the basis of the available evidence, there is no survival benefit for second-look laparotomy. Such procedures should only be undertaken as part of a clinical trial. Likewise, the value of secondary tumour resection at the time of second-look laparotomy remains unclear.

CURRENT STANDARD

Second-look laparotomy has no place in the routine management of women with ovarian carcinoma.

Interval debulking surgery

The concept of interval debulking surgery arose following the disappointing results achieved with second-look laparotomy. If initial maximal cytoreduction was not performed, interval debulking should be considered in patients responding to chemotherapy, or showing stable disease. Following the Goldie–Coldman model, interval debulking surgery should be performed as soon as chemotherapy has produced the necessary cytoreduction; usually after three cycles of chemotherapy, followed by three further cycles of chemotherapy.

There exist three prospective randomised trials regarding interval debulking surgery. The first was carried out in the West Midlands and included 79 patients with bulky residual disease after primary surgery.[25] They were randomised to either interval debulking surgery or standard chemotherapy alone. No significant difference in survival was found to justify the increased surgical morbidity. In the EORTC trial, 425 women were enrolled into the study, of whom 319 were subsequently randomised.[26] Women were eligible to enter if they had not been optimally debulked (greater than 1 cm residual tumour deposit). After three cycles of chemotherapy, and if they responded, they were randomised to interval debulking surgery or no further surgery. All randomised women received six cycles of platinum-based chemotherapy. Women in the interval debulking surgery arm demonstrated a 6-month median survival advantage ($P = 0.001$). The authors conclude that the increased morbidity was acceptable in view of the survival advantage. In contrast, a subsequent GOG randomised prospective trial (GOG 152) of 424 women showed no difference in median survival for women receiving interval debulking surgery.[27] The median survival for both the control arm and the interval debulking surgery arm was 36 months in the GOG study. In contrast, the EORTC demonstrated an overall survival of 26 months. The difference in survival is partly due to the use of carboplatin and paclitaxel in the GOG study compared to carboplatin and cyclophosphamide in the EORTC, a regimen that is now recognised as inferior. Furthermore, the overall patient population had been managed with more aggressive surgical approaches common in North American practice. The authors conclude that if the initial surgical debulking was undertaken by a gynaecological oncologist then interval debulking surgery is not recommended even if suboptimal debulking was achieved. The 10-year results of the EORTC study contain a persisting survival advantage in the interval debulking surgery arm. However, a Cochrane review could not conclude interval debulking surgery improves survival.[28]

CURRENT STANDARD

If initial maximal cytoreduction was not performed, interval debulking should be considered in patients responding to chemotherapy, or showing stable disease. If the initial surgical debulking was undertaken by a gynaecological oncologist then interval debulking surgery is not recommended, even if suboptimal debulking was achieved.

Neoadjuvant chemotherapy followed by surgery

A midline laparotomy is a major operation, with associated mortality and morbidity. Avoiding surgery for some patients may be beneficial in terms of survival and quality of life. Major complications of surgery include haemorrhage, infection, thromboembolic disease, wound dehiscence and bowel obstruction. Postoperative mortality after primary cytoreductive surgery is 3.7% on average and is more frequent for elderly women and after extensive procedures.[29] Neoadjuvant chemotherapy followed by surgery (NACT-S) is the term applied to the strategy of primary chemotherapy in potentially resectable cases. In this approach, patients with histologically or cytologically positive ovarian carcinoma are treated with primary chemotherapy before surgical debulking. This requires a reasonable certainty of the diagnosis, such as an ovarian mass, ascites or omental disease and an elevated serum CA125 level.

The EORTC randomised trial 55971 compared NACT-S with the standard primary surgery followed by platinum-based chemotherapy,[30] while the Medical Research Council CHORUS study is similar but with less stringent entry criteria.[31] Initial results of 55971 indicate that interval debulking surgery in this context is no less effective than up-front debulking but is less morbid and should be more widely considered than previously. CHORUS is still recruiting and the two trials should be added together for a final analysis.

CURRENT STANDARD

NACT-S should be offered to patients who are not fit for up-front surgical debulking or those in whom optimal debulking is unlikely.

First line chemotherapy for epithelial ovarian cancer

Although surgery is usually the primary treatment, ovarian cancer is a chemosensitive disease and chemotherapy has been shown to improve prognosis in advanced disease. Current guidelines recommend that chemotherapy is started no later than 8 weeks after initial surgery.

EARLY STAGE DISEASE

For optimally staged patients with FIGO stage Ia/b, well differentiated, non-clear cell histology surgery alone is adequate. ICON 1 (International Collaborative Ovarian Neoplasm)[32] and ACTION (Adjuvant ChemoTherapy in Ovarian Neoplasm)[33] trials have confirmed the survival advantage of adjuvant chemotherapy in early stage disease, with an 8% survival advantage at 6 years.[34] The recent Cochrane review showed an overall hazard ratio of 0.72 in favour of chemotherapy.[35] Thus, the majority of women who are assessed as having early-stage epithelial ovarian cancer will benefit from chemotherapy. The grade of the tumour is the most powerful prognostic indication in stage I disease and should be used in decision making in clinical practice.[36] Patients with FIGO stage Ia/b poorly differentiated, densely adherent, clear-cell histology and all grades FIGO stage Ic and IIa require optimal surgery and adjuvant chemotherapy should be considered.

Current standard

For patients with FIGO stage IA/B, well differentiated, non-clear-cell histology, surgery alone is adequate. FIGO stage IA/B poorly differentiated, densely adherent, clear-cell histology and all grades FIGO stage IC and IIA require optimal surgery and adjuvant chemotherapy.

ADVANCED DISEASE

For patients who are medically fit, the recommended standard primary chemotherapy for advanced ovarian carcinoma, stage Ic–IIIc, is carboplatin AUC (area under the concentration-time curve) 5–7 mg/ml/minute with paclitaxel 175 mg/m^2/3 hourly every 3 weeks for six cycles. This is based on two large positive trials, GOG III[37] and OV10.[38] Patients should receive optimal doses of chemotherapy based on measured glomerular filtration rate (GFR) and actual body weight; dose reductions for high body mass index (BMI) are discouraged. Patients are likely to experience more adverse effects with combined therapy compared with carboplatin alone and for these reasons it is not universally used as a first-line treatment. The decision to use combined or monotherapy will depend on the stage of the woman's disease, the extent of surgical treatment required and disease-related performance status. In such cases, the National Institute for Health and Clinical Excellence (NICE) advises treating with monotherapy (cisplatin or carboplatin).[39] Currently, in the UK, around 25% of patients are treated with single-agent carboplatin.

Recent trials, including ICON 5 and OV16, comparing three- and two-drug combinations have not shown any improvement over carboplatin and paclitaxel. The platinum agents remain the most effective agent with a benefit estimated at 2 months to 2 years. Current data do not support the recommendation of maintenance/consolidation treatment beyond six cycles.

Current standard

Standard chemotherapy for advanced ovarian carcinoma is carboplatin with or without paclitaxel every 3 weeks for six cycles. Current data do not support the recommendation of maintenance/consolidation treatment beyond six cycles.

INTRAPERITONEAL CHEMOTHERAPY

Several studies comparing different intravenous chemotherapy (cisplatin, paclitaxel) with intraperitoneal chemotherapy have shown improved survival in patients with optimally debulked stage III ovarian cancer.[40]

Morbidity, especially intraperitoneal catheter-related problems, pain, bowel obstruction and treatment-related mortality are significantly worse with intraperitoneal chemotherapy. Intraperitoneal chemotherapy has not been widely adopted, despite a National Cancer Institute announcement in 2006 recommending its implementation. However, selected patients with optimal tumour debulking and good performance status are likely to benefit from this treatment and it may, in time, gain acceptance. Intraperitoneal chemotherapy should be considered in centres where the expertise exists.

Current standard

Further trials are awaited. Intraperitoneal chemotherapy should be considered an option only in centres where the expertise exists.

NOVEL CHEMOTHERAPEUTIC AND BIOLOGICAL AGENTS

Novel chemotherapeutic agents are constantly being developed. Current avenues being pursued in ovarian cancer include hormonal therapies, anti-angiogenic drugs and growth factor inhibitors. Their main advantage is their minimal adverse effects when compared with conventional chemotherapy. Single-agent bevacizumab, a vascular endothelial growth factor (VEGF) inhibitor, has demonstrated significant clinical activity in multiple phase II studies. Translational studies are needed to help design rational combinations of targeted agents and to help predict response to therapy.

Management of relapsed disease

Unfortunately, for the majority of women with advanced disease, treatment will not be curative. Most women will show some level of response to primary chemotherapy but subsequent relapses are highly likely. Second- and third-line therapy in ovarian cancer is often hampered by the tumour's intrinsic or acquired resistance to platinum-based chemotherapy. Thus, treatment for relapsed disease is usually regarded as a palliative measure in women with symptomatic recurrent tumours.

THE ROLE OF CHEMOTHERAPY IN RECURRENT DISEASE

The choice of second-line treatment is determined by the tumour's level of platinum sensitivity, defined by NICE as:

- platinum-sensitive ovarian cancer: disease that responds to first-line platinum-based therapy but relapses 12 months or more after completion of initial platinum-based chemotherapy
- partially platinum-sensitive ovarian cancer: disease that responds to first-line platinum-based therapy but relapses between 6 and 12 months after completion of initial platinum-based chemotherapy
- platinum-resistant ovarian cancer: disease that relapses within 6 months of completion of initial platinum-based chemotherapy
- platinum-refractory ovarian cancer: disease that does not respond to initial platinum-based chemotherapy.[39]

The results of ICON 4 demonstrated a 3-month survival benefit and disease-free survival benefit for relapsed platinum-sensitive and partially sensitive disease treated with combination carboplatin/paclitaxel compared with single-agent carboplatin.[41] However, 75% of the patients had a platinum-free interval of 12 months or more. For platinum-sensitive recurrent tumours, a combination of paclitaxel and platinum-based therapy is recommended. Retreatment with paclitaxel is associated with a 20% incidence of G3/4 neuropathy, however, and this must be carefully considered when planning treatment. For tumours that are platinum-resistant, or platinum-refractory alternative chemotherapy drugs, pegylated liposomal doxorubicin hydrochloride (Caelyx®, Schering-Plough) and topotecan (Hycamtin®, GSK) may be considered.

Current practice

Patients with long intervals (over 6 months) from initial chemotherapy should be offered platinum-based combination chemotherapy (carboplatin + paclitaxel, carboplatin + gemcitabine). For patients with short treatment-free intervals (less than 6 months), chemotherapy with pegylated liposomal doxorubicin, gemcitabine or topotecan should be considered.

NOVEL CHEMOTHERAPEUTIC AGENTS

Novel chemotherapeutic agents are constantly being developed and include hormonal therapies, anti-angiogenic drugs and growth factor inhibitors. Hormonal therapies probably act by reducing estrogen activity and include tamoxifen, aromatase inhibitors and gonadotrophin-releasing hormone analogues. Response rates of 10–15% have been achieved in relapsed disease. Their main advantage is their minimal adverse effects when compared with conventional chemotherapy. One of the most promising developments is the monoclonal antibody to VEGF, bevacizumab. VEGF is an important factor in neoangiogenesis and a poor prognostic feature in ovarian cancer. Bevacizumab is already in use for advanced bowel carcinoma and renal-cell carcinoma. Early studies in ovarian cancer are promising, although there are concerns about an increased risk of bowel perforation. A large phase III trial of bevacizumab with carboplatin and paclitaxel after surgical debulking (ICON 7) is currently underway.

THE ROLE OF SURGERY IN RELAPSED DISEASE

The role of surgery in recurrent ovarian cancer is still being developed. There are at present no randomised controlled trials but the consensus supports aggressive surgical debulking for patients with:

- prolonged disease-free survival (12–18 months)
- solitary or a limited number of sites of recurrence
- good performance status
- absence of ascites.

These are similar to the prognostic indicators for second-line chemotherapy.

Imaging is insensitive with up to 50% of the women, with single-site recurrence on CT being found to have carcinomatosis or multiple sites of tumour on subsequent laparotomy. A large, retrospective review of surgery in 267 women with recurrent disease was recently reported. The DESKTOP trial[42] was a retrospective exploratory study based on women treated in 25 collaborating institutions from 2000 to 2003. Complete resection was associated with significantly longer survival compared with those in whom any macroscopic disease remained (median 45.2 months compared with 19.7 months; hazard ratio 3.71; 95% confidence interval 2.27–6.05; $P < .0001$). Interestingly, the size of macroscopic tumour had no impact on survival. Variables associated with complete resection were performance status, FIGO stage at initial diagnosis and absence of ascites greater than 500 ml. A combination of: performance status, early initial FIGO stage or no residual tumour after first surgery and absence of ascites could predict complete resection in 79% of patients.

Only complete resection was associated with prolonged survival in recurrent ovarian cancer. These findings are interesting but, being based on retrospective data, figures should be interpreted with caution. The identified criteria panel will be verified in a prospective trial (Arbeitsgemeinschaft Gynaekologische Onkologie [AGO] DESKTOP II OVAR 3) evaluating whether it will render a useful tool for selecting the right patients for cytoreductive surgery in recurrent ovarian cancer.

CURRENT PRACTICE

We await phase III studies to address this issue fully (AGO DESKTOP OVAR II and GOG 213).

Patients with a long interval (longer than 1 year) from primary surgery should, however, be considered for surgical resection of recurrent disease.

Radiotherapy

Radiotherapy has a more limited role, primarily in palliation of advanced disease. This includes the control of pain, which is most often caused by metastatic bone disease or lymphadenopathy, and the control of vaginal bleeding.

CURRENT PRACTICE

Radiotherapy is mainly used as a palliative treatment to reduce pain and, occasionally, to control bleeding.

Minimal access surgery

Although minimal-access surgery is frequently being used for benign ovarian cysts, inappropriate treatment of malignant tumours by laparoscopic resection is associated with the risk of disease spreading throughout the abdominal cavity.[43] The role of minimal-access surgery in the management of ovarian carcinoma has yet to be properly defined. However, it is increasingly being used for obtaining tissue for histological diagnosis and staging, particularly in assessing patients for surgery in recurrent disease.

CURRENT PRACTICE

The role of minimal-access surgery in the management of ovarian carcinoma has yet to be properly defined.

Response evaluation

In women whose tumours are secretors, the level of serum CA125 during chemotherapy correlates with tumour response and with their overall survival.[44] Serum CA125 should be measured at regular intervals during chemotherapy. For women with an abnormal CT at base line, this should be repeated after six cycles of chemotherapy unless there is clinical or biochemical evidence of progressive disease (such as persistent ascites or serum CA125 not falling), when the CT scan should be repeated earlier. Women with a normal CT at baseline do not need a further CT scan unless it is clinically indicated. However, for women who are non-secretors (negative for serum CA125) a CT scan should be performed after three cycles to assess response to chemotherapy. In addition, those women who are being considered for interval debulking surgery should have a CT scan after three cycles; the scan should be discussed in the multidisciplinary team meeting.

CURRENT STANDARD

Serum CA125 should be measured at regular intervals during chemotherapy. A CT scan should be considered after 3–6 months, depending on response to chemotherapy and before interval debulking surgery.

Follow-up

The primary aims of routine follow-up are to identify disease recurrence before symptoms occur, to provide psychological support and reassurance and symptom control related to treatment and the cancer. Data on survival and recurrence are also collected. The absence of symptoms, however, does not indicate the absence of recurrent disease. Approximately 40% of women with no clinical or ultrasound evidence of disease are found to have disease at second-look laparotomy.[45] Furthermore, the process of attending clinics, undergoing CT scans and blood tests and awaiting results of investigations generates anxiety. There is no standard follow-up protocol for any of the gynaecological cancers; however, follow-up investigations continue to be standard practice, despite limited evidence to support their use.[46] Current practice is to follow up every 3–4 months in the first 2 years and to reduce that to 6-monthly intervals for 3–5 years or until progression is documented. At each appointment, a history should be taken and a physical examination, including pelvic examination, should be performed. CT scans should be performed if there is clinical evidence of progressive disease.

Serum CA125 can accurately predict tumour recurrence and often increases several months before the patient is symptomatic or has measurable disease. The MRC/EORTC sponsored OV05/55955 study involved the randomisation of patients to immediate treatment with a rising serum CA125 level or waiting until the patient was symptomatic; 527 patients were randomised from 1442 registered in ten countries: 264 patients started second-line chemotherapy a median of 5 months earlier in the immediate arm. There was no difference in overall survival between the immediate and delayed arms (hazard ratio 1.01, 95% confidence interval 0.82–1.25, $P = 0.91$). The authors concluded that there was no value in the routine measurement of serum CA125 in the follow-up of women with ovarian cancer.[47] Radiological examination, such as CT, has not been shown to improve the detection of recurrence. Fluorodeoxyglucose-PET scans may be superior in detecting small volume operable relapses.

Women with a family history

Whereas women with no family history of ovarian cancer have a 1.5% lifetime risk of developing the disease, those with one affected first-degree relative (mother, daughter, sister) have a 5% risk and women with two first-degree relatives have a 7% risk. The risk is somewhat lower for women with one first-degree and one second-degree relative (grandmother, aunt) with ovarian cancer (Table 9.2). Overall, approximately 5–10 % of cases of ovarian cancer are thought to be familial. It has become well established that inherited mutations in either *BRCA1* or *BRCA2* confer Mendelian dominant genetic predisposition to both breast and ovarian cancer, with approximately 80% penetrance. *BRCA1* is found in 5% of women diagnosed with ovarian cancer before the age of 70 years. Unfortunately, this is a large gene with over 100 000 base pairs, any one of which may be mutated. Estimates of the lifetime cancer risk associated with *BRCA* mutations are variable and depend upon the population studied, ranging from 15–60% for ovarian cancer, compared with a 1.5% lifetime risk among the general population.[5] There are likely to be several genes that predispose to ovarian cancer, some associated with colon cancer syndromes such as hereditary non-polyposis colorectal cancer (HNPCC) also known as Lynch type II. HNPCC is known to slightly increase the risk of developing ovarian cancer; associated lifetime risk is 9 to 12%.

The genetic predisposition for an individual woman can be difficult to determine without expert knowledge. Multiple primary cancers in one individual or related early-onset cancers in a family tree are suggestive of a predisposing gene. Except for those families where a specific gene abnormality is identifiable, there are few families in which it is possible to be sure of dominant inheritance but where four first-degree relatives have early-onset or bilateral breast cancer in combination with ovarian cancer, the risk of inheriting a mutated gene is close to 50%.

Table 9.2	Approximate lifetime percentage risk of developing ovarian cancer
Population	*Lifetime risk (%)*
General	1.5
one first-degree relative affected under 55 years	5.2
one first-degree relative affected over 55 years	3.4
two first-degree relatives affected	7
BRCA1 carrier	28–44
BRCA2 carrier	27
HNPCC carrier	12

Careful family history and referral to the cancer genetics team should follow locally agreed guidelines. Individuals assessed to be at increased risk of ovarian cancer may be offered annual transvaginal ovarian ultrasound and serum CA125 tumour marker blood test. Screening should start at age 30 years or 5 years before the age of onset of the first ovarian cancer in the family. Once their family is complete, prophylactic risk-reducing surgery is recommended for *BRCA1* and *BRCA2* carriers. For oophorectomy, a prospective study of 170 women found that the risk of cancer was reduced from 6.9% to 3.1% after a mean period of 2 years.[48] Surgery usually consists of laparoscopic bilateral salpingo-oophorectomy, while HNPCC carriers are also offered hysterectomy. Neither prophylactic surgery nor screening can completely eliminate the possibility of developing cancer. Screening is not proven to improve survival and, even if the ovaries are removed, there is a small continuing risk of developing primary peritoneal cancer. The United Kingdom Familial Ovarian Cancer Screening Study (UKFOCSS) aimed to recruit 5000 women aged 35 years or over and will assess whether regular screening is beneficial for women at high risk of developing ovarian cancer. Recruitment closed in December 2009. Women participating in the trial will have a serum CA125 test three times a year for up to 4 years and transvaginal ultrasound once a year for up to 4 years. This trial is expected to report in 2012.

CURRENT STANDARD

Women with a family history that appears to place them at high risk of developing ovarian cancer (Box 9.1) should be offered referral to a clinical genetics service for assessment and confirmation of their family history.

BOX. 9.1 CRITERIA FOR CATEGORISATION OF A WOMAN AS AT HIGH RISK OF OVARIAN CANCER

- Two or more first-degree relatives affected by ovarian cancer.
- One first-degree relative with ovarian cancer and one with breast cancer diagnosed before the age of 50 years. One first-degree relative with ovarian cancer and two with breast cancer diagnosed before the age of 60 years.
- An individual with a mutation of one of the genes known to predispose to ovarian cancer.
- Three first-degree relatives with colorectal cancer with at least one diagnosed below the age of 50 years, as well as one case of ovarian cancer.

They may then be eligible for referral for screening via a research trial and/or offered prophylactic surgery.

Screening for ovarian carcinoma

Unfortunately, borderline ovarian tumours rarely precede invasive tumours; thus, the identification of a premalignant stage in ovarian cancer has yet to be identified. The multicentre United Kingdom Collaborative Trial of Ovarian Cancer Screening (UKCTOCS) is the largest study of its kind to date: 202 638 postmenopausal women aged 50–74 years were randomised to no treatment (control group), annual multimodal screening of transvaginal ultrasound and serum CA125 and transvaginal ultrasound alone in a 2:1:1 ratio. Menon *et al.*[49] reported on the sensitivity and specificity of the prevalence screen. On the initial screen, 58 invasive ovarian and fallopian tube cancers were detected in the screening groups, of which 24 (14 multimodal screening, 10 ultrasound) were stage I. However, 35 surgeries for invasive cancer had to be performed in the ultrasound group compared with 2.9 in the multimodal screening group. The prevalence screen has established that the screening strategies are feasible; however, we will have to wait to see whether screening has an effect on mortality when the trial is concluded in 2014. It also aims to comprehensively address the cost, acceptance, physical and psychological morbidity. Until then, there is no indication to screen for ovarian carcinoma in women without a familial history of ovarian and breast cancer.

CURRENT STANDARD

There is no indication to screen for ovarian carcinoma in women without a familial history of ovarian and breast cancer. Results from the current UKCTOCS trial are not expected until 2014.

Reference List

1. Berrino F, De AR, Sant M, Rosso S, Bielska-Lasota M, Coebergh JW, *et al.* Survival for eight major cancers and all cancers combined for European adults diagnosed in 1995–99: results of the EUROCARE-4 study. *Lancet Oncol* 2007;8:773–83.

2. Ferlay J, Bray F, Pisani P, Parkin DM. GLOBOCAN 2002. *Cancer Incidence, Mortality and Prevalence Worldwide. IARC Cancer Base No. 5, Version 2.0.* Lyon: IARC Press; 2004.

3. Parkin DM, Bray F, Ferlay J, Pisani P. Global cancer statistics, 2002. *CA Cancer J Clin* 2005;55:74–108.

4. Kirwan JM, Tincello DG, Herod JJ, Frost O, Kingston RE. Effect of delays in primary care referral on survival of women with epithelial ovarian cancer: retrospective audit. *BMJ* 2002;324:148–51.

5. Cancer Research UK. *CancerStats report: Ovarian Cancer UK.* London: Cancer Research UK; 2004.

6. de Nictolis M, Montironi R, Tommasoni S, Carinelli S, Ojeda B, Matías-Guiu X, *et al.* Serous borderline tumors of the ovary: a clinicopathologic, immunohisto-chemical, and quantitative study of 44 cases. *Cancer* 2006;70:152–60.

7. Colombo N, Parma G, Zanagnolo V, Insinga A. Management of ovarian stromal cell tumors. *J Clin Oncol* 2007;25:2944–51.

8. Gershenson DM. Management of ovarian germ cell tumors. *J Clin Oncol* 2007;25:2938–43.

9. Flam F, Einhorn N, Sjovall K. Symptomatology of ovarian cancer. *Eur J Obstet Gynecol Reprod Biol* 1988;27:53–7.

10. Goff BA, Mandel LS, Drescher CW, Urban N, Gough S, Schurman KM, *et al.* Development of an ovarian cancer symptom index: possibilities for earlier detection. *Cancer* 2007;109:221–7.

11. Davies AP, Jacobs I, Woolas R, Fish A, Oram D. The adnexal mass: benign or malignant? Evaluation of a risk of malignancy index. *Br J Obstet Gynaecol* 1993;100:927–31.

12. Goncalves V, Jayson G, Tarrier N. A longitudinal investigation of psychological morbidity in patients with ovarian cancer. *Br J Cancer* 2008;99:1794–801.

13. Kavanagh JJ, Pecorelli S, Benedetti JL. Cancer of the ovary. In: Pecorelli S, Ngan HYS, Hacker NF, editors. *Staging Classifications and Clinical Practice. Guidelines for Gynaecological Cancers.* 3rd ed. London: International Federation of Gynecology and Obstetrics; 2000. p. 95–121.

14. Current FIGO staging for cancer of the vagina, fallopian tube, ovary, and gestational trophoblastic neoplasia. *Int J Gynecol Obstet* 2009;105:3–4.

15. Griffiths CT. Surgical resection of tumor bulk in the primary treatment of ovarian carcinoma. *Natl Cancer Inst Monogr* 1975;42:101–4.

16. Bristow RE, Tomacruz RS, Armstrong DK, Trimble EL, Montz FJ. Survival effect of maximal cytoreductive surgery for advanced ovarian carcinoma during the platinum era: a meta-analysis. *J Clin Oncol* 2002;20:1248–59.

17. Winter WE III, Maxwell GL, Tian C, Carlson JW, Ozols RF, Rose PG, *et al.* Prognostic factors for stage III epithelial ovarian cancer: a Gynecologic Oncology Group Study. *J Clin Oncol* 2007;25:3621–7.

18. Eisenhauer EL, Abu-Rustum NR, Sonoda Y, Aghajanian C, Barakat RR, Chi DS. The effect of maximal surgical cytoreduction on sensitivity to platinum-taxane chemotherapy and subsequent survival in patients with advanced ovarian cancer. *Gynecol Oncol* 2008;108:276–81.

19. Winter WE III, Maxwell GL, Tian C, Sundborg MJ, Rose GS, Rose PG, *et al.* Tumor residual after surgical cytoreduction in prediction of clinical outcome in stage IV epithelial ovarian cancer: a Gynecologic Oncology Group Study. *J Clin Oncol* 2008;26:83–9.

20. Eisenkop SM, Spirtos NM, Friedman RL, Lin WC, Pisani AL, Perticucci S. Relative influences of tumor volume before surgery and the cytoreductive outcome on survival for patients with advanced ovarian cancer: a prospective study. *Gynecol Oncol* 2003;90:390–6.

21. Eisenkop SM, Friedman RL, Wang HJ. Complete cytoreductive surgery is feasible and maximizes survival in patients with advanced epithelial ovarian cancer: a prospective study. *Gynecol Oncol* 1998;69:103–8.

22. Scholz HS, Tasdemir H, Hunlich T, Turnwald W, Both A, Egger H. Multivisceral cytoreductive surgery in FIGO stages IIIC and IV epithelial ovarian cancer: results and 5-year follow-up. *Gynecol Oncol* 2007;106:591–5.

23. Panici PB, Maggioni A, Hacker N, Landoni F, Ackermann S, Campagnutta E, *et al*. Systematic aortic and pelvic lymphadenectomy versus resection of bulky nodes only in optimally debulked advanced ovarian cancer: a randomized clinical trial. *J Natl Cancer Inst* 2005;97:560–6.

24. Jemal A, Siegel R, Ward E, Hao Y, Xu J, Thun MJ. Cancer Statistics, 2009. *CA Cancer J Clin* 2009;59:225–49.

25. Redman CW, Warwick J, Luesley DM, Varma R, Lawton FG, Blackledge GR. Intervention debulking surgery in advanced epithelial ovarian cancer. *Br J Obstet Gynaecol* 1994;101:142–6.

26. van der Burg ME, van Lent M, Buyse M, Kobierska A, Colombo N, Favalli G, *et al*. The effect of debulking surgery after induction chemotherapy on the prognosis in advanced epithelial ovarian cancer. Gynecological Cancer Cooperative Group of the European Organization for Research and Treatment of Cancer. *N Engl J Med* 1995;332:629–34.

27. Rose PG, Nerenstone S, Brady MF, Clarke-Pearson D, Olt G, Rubin SC, *et al*. Secondary surgical cytoreduction for advanced ovarian carcinoma. *N Engl J Med* 2004;351:2489–97.

28. Tangjitgamol S, Manusirivithaya S, Laopaiboon M, Lumbiganon P. Interval debulking surgery for advanced epithelial ovarian cancer: a Cochrane systematic review. *Gynecol Oncol* 2009 Jan;112(1):257-64.

29. Gerestein CG, Damhuis RA, Burger CW, Kooi GS. Postoperative mortality after primary cytoreductive surgery for advanced stage epithelial ovarian cancer: a systematic review. *Gynecol Oncol* 2009;114:523–7.

30. European Organisation for Research and Treatment of Cancer Gynaecological Cancer Group. EORTC 55971: a randomized phase III study comparing upfront debulking surgery vs neo-adjuvant chemotherapy in patients with stage IIIc or IV epithelial ovarian carcinoma. Dr Sergio Pecorelli, Professor Gordon Rustin, Ignace Vergote [http://groups.eortc.be/gcg/studyprotocols.htm#55971].

31. Phase II/III randomized pilot study of the timing of surgery and chemotherapy in patients with newly diagnosed advanced ovarian epithelial, fallopian tube, or primary peritoneal cavity cancer [www.cancer.gov/clinicaltrials/RCOG-MRC-CHORUS].

32. Colombo N, Guthrie D, Chiari S, Parmar M, Qian W, Swart AM, *et al*. International Collaborative Ovarian Neoplasm trial 1: a randomized trial of adjuvant chemotherapy in women with early-stage ovarian cancer. *J Natl Cancer Inst* 2003;95:125–32.

33. Trimbos JB, Vergote I, Bolis G, Vermorken JB, Mangioni C, Madronal C, *et al*. Impact of adjuvant chemotherapy and surgical staging in early-stage ovarian carcinoma: European Organisation for Research and Treatment of Cancer Adjuvant ChemoTherapy in Ovarian Neoplasm trial. *J Natl Cancer Inst* 2003;95:113–25.

34. Trimbos JB, Parmar M, Vergote I, Guthrie D, Bolis G, Colombo N, *et al*. International Collaborative Ovarian Neoplasm trial 1 and Adjuvant ChemoTherapy In Ovarian Neoplasm trial: two parallel randomized phase III trials of adjuvant chemotherapy in patients with early-stage ovarian carcinoma. *J Natl Cancer Inst* 2003;95:105–12.

35. Winter-Roach BA, Kitchener HC, Dickinson HO. Adjuvant (post-surgery) chemotherapy for early stage epithelial ovarian cancer. *Cochrane Database Syst Rev* 2009;(1):CD004706.

36. Vergote I, De BJ, Fyles A, Bertelsen K, Einhorn N, Sevelda P, *et al*. Prognostic importance of degree of differentiation and cyst rupture in stage I invasive epithelial ovarian carcinoma. *Lancet* 2001;357:176–82.

37. McGuire WP, Hoskins WJ, Brady MF, Kucera PR, Partridge EE, Look KY, *et al*. Cyclophosphamide and cisplatin compared with paclitaxel and cisplatin in patients with stage III and stage IV ovarian cancer. *N Engl J Med* 1996;334:1–6.

38. Piccart MJ, Bertelsen K, James K, Cassidy J, Mangioni C, Simonsen E, *et al*. Randomized intergroup trial of cisplatin-paclitaxel versus cisplatin-cyclophosphamide in women with advanced epithelial ovarian cancer: three-year results. *J Natl Cancer Inst* 2000;92:699–708.

39. Main C, Bojke L, Griffin S, Norman G, Barbieri M, Mather L, *et al*. Topotecan, pegylated liposomal doxorubicin hydrochloride and paclitaxel for second-line or subsequent treatment of advanced ovarian cancer: a systematic review and economic evaluation. *Health Technol Assess* 2006;10(9):1–132.

40. Armstrong DK, Bundy B, Wenzel L, Huang HQ, Baergen R, Lele S, *et al*. Intraperitoneal cisplatin and paclitaxel in ovarian cancer. *N Engl J Med* 2006;354:34–43.

41. Parmar MK, Ledermann JA, Colombo N, du BA, Delaloye JF, Kristensen GB, *et al*. Paclitaxel plus platinum-based chemotherapy versus conventional platinum-based chemotherapy in women with relapsed ovarian cancer: the ICON4/AGO-OVAR-2.2 trial. *Lancet* 2003;361:2099–106.

42. Harter P, du Bois A, Hahmann M, Hasenburg A, Burges A, Loibl S, *et al*. Surgery in recurrent ovarian cancer: the Arbeitsgemeinschaft Gynaekologische Onkologie (AGO) DESKTOP OVAR trial. *Ann Surg Oncol* 2006;13:1702–10.

43. Medeiros LR, Rosa DD, Bozzetti MC, Fachel JM, Furness S, Garry R, *et al*. Laparoscopy versus laparotomy for benign ovarian tumour. *Cochrane Database Syst Rev* 2009;(2):CD004751.

44. Rustin GJ, Nelstrop AE, McClean P, Brady MF, McGuire WP, Hoskins WJ, *et al*. Defining response of ovarian carcinoma to initial chemotherapy according to serum CA 125. *J Clin Oncol* 1996;14:1545–51.

45. Bristow RE, Lagasse LD, Karlan BY. Secondary surgical cytoreduction for advanced epithelial ovarian cancer. Patient selection and review of the literature. *Cancer* 1996;78:2049–62.

46. Kew FM, Cruickshank DJ. Routine follow-up after treatment for a gynecological cancer: a survey of practice. *Int J Gynecol Cancer* 2006;16:380–4.

47. Rustin GJ, van der Burg ME, on behalf of MRC and EORTC collaborators. A randomized trial in ovarian cancer (OC) of early treatment of relapse based on CA125 level alone versus delayed treatment based on conventional clinical indicators (MRC OV05/EORTC 55955 trials). *Int J Clin Oncol* 2009;27 Suppl:18.

48. Kauff ND, Satagopan JM, Robson ME, Scheuer L, Hensley M, Hudis CA, *et al*. Risk-reducing salpingo-oophorectomy in women with a BRCA1 or BRCA2 mutation. *N Engl J Med* 2002;346:1609–15.

49. Menon U, Gentry-Maharaj A, Hallett R, Ryan A, Burnell M, Sharma A, *et al.* Sensitivity and specificity of multimodal and ultrasound screening for ovarian cancer, and stage distribution of detected cancers: results of the prevalence screen of the UK Collaborative Trial of Ovarian Cancer Screening (UKCTOCS). *Lancet Oncol* 2009;10:327–40.

10 Endometrial cancer standards of care

Signs and symptoms

Postmenopausal bleeding is the most common complaint in women in whom endometrial cancer is diagnosed. Around 90% of women are diagnosed after the age of 50 years and postmenopausal bleeding is associated with an underlying carcinoma in up to 10% of women. While commonly associated with older women, endometrial cancer can occur in younger women and may present with irregular or intermenstrual bleeding. Such women often experience a delay in diagnosis, as management may initially be via a menstrual disorders clinic and characteristic findings at hysteroscopy may be lacking. Because of the strong aetiological association with estrogenic stimulation, the diagnosis should be considered in symptomatic younger women with polycystic ovary syndrome, those with irregular bleeding on hormone replacement therapy or those taking tamoxifen. Tamoxifen stimulates ovarian estrogen biosynthesis and elevates plasma estrogen levels, increasing the risk of endometrial cancer.

Endometrial hyperplasia can be termed a premalignant condition of the endometrium. Occurring as a result of estrogenic stimulation of the endometrium, endometrial hyperplasia is classified as simple or complex – in the absence of cytological atypia the risk of malignancy is low (1–4%) but the risk of co-existing or rapidly developing malignancy with a histological finding of complex endometrial hyperplasia with atypia may be as high as 43%.

Two distinct forms of endometrial cancer were described by Bohkman in 1983 and these distinct types are recognised when planning clinical management. Type 1 endometrial cancer is the most common, with over 80% of cases. The common risk factors are often found in women who are over-weight who develop grade 1–2, often superficially, invasive cancers. Type 1 endometrial cancer often arises in association with atypical endometrial hyperplasia. Such cases are usually associated with a 5-year survival of around 85%.

Type 2 endometrial cancers are not associated with estrogenic stimulation and include variants such as serous, clear-cell, small-cell, carcinosarcoma and other rare subtypes. Such cases metastasise early and carry a much poorer prognosis, with a 50% 5-year survival.

In addition to these subtypes, a variety of smooth-muscle tumours can arise in the uterus. These range from the very common and benign leiomyoma (fibroid), through to malignant tumours such as carcinosarcoma or leiomyosarcoma. Carcinosarcomas are also known as malignant mixed müllerian tumours. Malignant smooth-muscle tumours of the uterus are uncommon, accounting for less than 5% of uterine tumours. It is estimated that the risk of malignant change in a fibroid is of the order of 1%, with rapid increase in the size of a fibroid a worrying sign that malignant transformation of a fibroid may be occurring.

While hysterectomy and bilateral salpingo-oophorectomy remains the mainstay of treatment, significant challenges remain to individualise staging and adjuvant therapy to improve the outcomes particularly for the poor prognostic subtypes, where a high risk of distant metastases and recurrence exists.

Investigation

Women presenting with postmenopausal bleeding are at risk of having endometrial cancer and investigations to confirm or exclude such a possibility should be performed (see also Chapter 4). As the risk of having cancer is approximately 10%, these women should be referred for gynaecological assessment at a local cancer unit, where there is a gynaecologist with a special interest in gynaecological oncology.

Many women with postmenopausal bleeding will not require an urgent assessment but they should be given an early appointment. Those at increased risk of cancer should be seen within 2 weeks of their general practitioner's referral.

Clinical history is important in putting into context the result of triage investigations. These are often performed on an outpatient basis and, in many units, dedicated rapid access clinics have been established to investigate postmenopausal bleeding. Transvaginal ultrasound is commonly used as a screening tool to assess the endometrial thickness. If the overall thickness of the endometrium is 4 mm or less and the ovaries appear normal on the scan, the probability of endometrial cancer is low. The pre-test risk of endometrial cancer for those with postmenopausal bleeding is reduced from 10% to 1% in those with a normal transvaginal scan. In cases of a single light bleed in the presence of negative cervical pathology, this may be the only investigation undertaken.[1,2]

Endometrial biopsies can be obtained as an outpatient using a variety of sampling devices. Some units use outpatient hysteroscopy as the screening investigation, combined with endometrial biopsy if indicated. In cases where pathology is suspected or if the outpatient biopsy is unsatisfactory, inpatient hysteroscopy combined with dilatation and curettage is performed.[3,4]

Once the histological diagnosis is confirmed, minimum further investigations include a chest X-ray, full blood count and biochemical profile. Staging of endometrial cancer is based on surgicopathological findings rather than preoperative staging by examination under anaesthesia in contrast to cervical carcinoma. The role of cross-sectional imaging with magnetic resonance imaging (MRI) or computed tomography (CT) scanning remains controversial. The potential benefits of MRI are in the prediction of depth of myometrial invasion, the presence of cervical involvement or extrauterine disease and identification of pelvic or para-aortic lymphadenopathy. (Figure 10.1) CT imaging allows greater assessment of possible distant metastases as well as identifying pelvic and para-aortic lymphadenopathy. It could be argued that hysteroscopy is a better method of assessing the endocervix and clinical impression of an endometrial rather than cervical primary cancer a more accurate

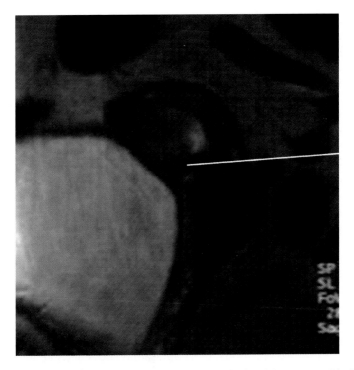

Figure 10.1 MRI of the uterus showing an anterior fundal tumour with deep myometrial extension (loss of the junctional zone)

discriminator. While MRI may allow identification of women with deep myometrial invasion, this may prove more difficult with high-grade tumours or in the presence of benign pathology, such as fibroids, in causing distortion of the junctional zone.[5,6] The other important issue continues to be the additional interventional decisions that such information allows. The preoperative identification of pelvic or para-aortic lymphadenopathy is potentially useful in allowing selective node sampling, which would impact on the decisions around adjuvant therapy. For laparoscopic management, it is also helpful to have an accurate indication of uterine size.

The original staging system introduced by FIGO in 1988 has been revised to focus on factors likely to change adjuvant management decisions and influence outcomes (see Appendix 1).

Surgical management

The standard surgical procedure for the management of endometrial cancer is hysterectomy and bilateral salpingo-oophorectomy by a method that allows evaluation of the peritoneal cavity. Traditionally, this would be performed by laparotomy via a lower midline incision. However, with large studies demonstrating comparable outcomes and enhanced recovery, best practice would now be via laparoscopically assisted or total laparoscopic hysterectomy.[7] This allows direct inspection of the peritoneum, omentum and liver and can be combined with pelvic lymphadenectomy or sampling, depending on the preoperative management decision. Even in women who have asymptomatic distant disease identified on preoperative imaging, a decision to proceed with hysterectomy and bilateral salpingo-oophorec-tomy may be made for local control and management of vaginal bleeding.

The role of lymphadenectomy in the management of endometrial cancer has been the subject of much debate with differing standard practices internationally and significant variations with UK gynaecological cancer centres. While full surgical staging by performing pelvic and para-aortic lymphadenectomy improves knowledge of extent of disease and thus the options for adjuvant therapy, it cannot be performed without consideration of the additional therapeutic benefit that any such interventions allow.

The risk of locoregional pelvic nodal recurrence and distant recurrence can be estimated from knowledge of the grade and depth of myometrial invasion. Well-differentiated cancers with superficial invasion only may have a rate of pelvic node involvement of 5% or less. However, in those women with poorly differentiated tumours and deep myometrial invasion studies have shown a 30% rate of pelvic nodal disease and a 30% rate of distant recurrence at 5 years, even after adjuvant pelvic radiotherapy at initial treatment.[8,9,10] Supporters of extended surgical staging by including para-aortic lymphadenectomy would point to recurrence in the para-aortic nodes that had not been adequately staged at initial surgery. The extent of para-aortic lymphadenectomy required is not well defined and evidence is lacking to show improved survival with currently available adjuvant therapy in patients who are node positive.[11,12]

Large retrospective non-randomised historical trials from the USA have suggested some survival benefit in pelvic lymph-node sampling which was further enhanced by systematic lymphadenectomy.[13] Such trials, however, contained multiple selection and treatment inconsistencies. The role of extended surgical staging and adjuvant pelvic radiotherapy was addressed by the ASTEC trial with a double randomisation to pelvic lymphadenectomy and pelvic radiotherapy possible in patients with a high risk of disease.[14] The study results were criticised for variations in surgical technique and in the extent of lymphadenectomy but no positive benefit was seen in life expectancy for those patients undergoing extending surgical staging as a therapeutic procedure or when combined with adjuvant pelvic radio-therapy. The theory that removal of microscopic disease present in pelvic nodes would have therapeutic benefit (extrapolated from lymphadenec-tomy in cervical cancer as part of radical hysterectomy) was not supported by the ASTEC findings. Moreover, those who had a more extensive lymphadenectomy did not show any difference in outcome but had more significant complications. Similar findings were reported in a further prospective randomised trial by Panici.[15]

Equally important is avoidance of adverse effects from surgical treatment and radiotherapy in patients at low risk of recurrence. Pelvic lymphadenectomy is associated with lower limb lymphoedema in 5–10% and vascular injury in 0.5–1.0%. The risk of lymphoedema increases with postoperative radiotherapy.[16]

Radiotherapy and chemotherapy

Women with endometrial cancer should be treated by surgery whenever possible. However, in those who are medically unfit with locally advanced disease, palliative radiotherapy to control vaginal bleeding is an option. The main role of radiotherapy is as adjuvant therapy. This may include external-beam pelvic treatment combined with vaginal brachytherapy. Despite initial evidence to the contrary,[17] it is now generally accepted that radiotherapy does not improve life expectancy and that its main role is in reducing the incidence of local recurrence. The most common site for local recurrence is at the vaginal vault and, overall, the risk is 15–20%. This risk may be halved by adjuvant brachytherapy.[18] If, however, a close observation policy is followed and local vault recurrence is detected early then salvage rates of 80% have been reported.

There is wide variability between centres in the use of adjuvant radiotherapy and no consensus on which patients should receive this type of treatment or on the type of radiotherapy (external beam, vault brachytherapy or both) that should be given. The majority of UK practice is to base decisions on the need for radiotherapy on the grade and depth of myometrial invasion with factors such as the presence of adverse factors (for example, lymphovascular invasion) taken into account. This is independent of histological assessment of the pelvic or para-aortic nodes.

While radiotherapy has not shown any survival benefit, it has been shown to have lasting adverse effects, including damage to the vagina, bowel and urinary tract. The combination of radiotherapy and surgery (particularly lymphadenectomy) may cause lymphoedema of the legs and lower abdomen. Disease-related deaths are often associated with failure to control recurrent distal disease, which, in most instances, is not related to pelvic disease control.

No evidence has been identified to suggest that primary or adjuvant chemotherapy improves survival for women with endometrial cancer. Systemic chemotherapy has typically been reserved for women with disseminated primary disease or extrapelvic recurrence. The use of chemotherapy is increasing particularly in non-endometrioid forms of endometrial cancer, particularly clear-cell and papillary serous, by extrapolation of evidence from treatment of ovarian carcinoma. There is no standard regimen but platinum–taxane combinations are most frequently used. The spread patterns are often different, with a higher incidence of extrauterine and distant disease. This needs to be balanced against the recorded potentially severe adverse effects. Patients with clear-cell or papillary serous tumours may receive pelvic radiotherapy and adjuvant chemotherapy to try to impact on the possibility of extrapelvic relapse. There may be a place for lymphadenectomy in such patients to be able to omit external beam therapy and consider adjuvant chemotherapy alone. However, there are no large trials to support this approach. It is hoped that trials such as PORTEC3, investigating the role of radiotherapy with chemotherapy, will address these issues.

Given the association with estrogen in the development of the more common variants of endometrial cancer, progestogens have traditionally been used as adjuvant therapy. However, a meta-analysis of the results of seven randomised controlled trials has shown that adjuvant progestogen therapy confers no survival benefit.[19] Progestogens should not therefore be used routinely for adjuvant treatment for endometrial cancer. In some women with progestogen receptor-positive recurrent tumours, there may be a role for a trial of therapy. Likewise, tamoxifen and other oral chemotherapy drugs commonly used for breast cancer hormone manipulations have shown disappointing results. The role of estrogen replacement remains controversial. In early-stage disease, there is probably no increased risk of relapse and therefore estrogen replacement could be considered in selected cases.

Palliative treatment and care

As with any cancer, women with advanced endometrial cancer, whether in hospital or in the community, should have access to specialist palliative care on a 24-hour basis and there should be local arrangements to ensure continuity of care. The aim of palliative care is to maintain and improve quality of life and the whole person should always be considered. It is important to provide both optimum relief from symptoms and to maintain the social and psychological wellbeing of the woman. Particular attention should be given to adequate pain control, for which effective interventions should be readily available. A variety of interventions, ranging from surgery to supportive care, may be necessary to improve quality of life for women going through the late stages of cancer. Patients and their relatives should be given realistic information about potential benefits, limitations and adverse effects of interventions and their views should always be respected. Most women with advancing cancer are likely to wish to remain at home for much of the duration of their illness. Women should be helped to remain in the place they prefer, whether this is their home, hospital or hospice, and should, whenever possible, be allowed to choose where they wish to die. Palliative aspects of care are addressed in more detail in Chapter 14.

Post-treatment support and follow-up

At present, there is no evidence to support routine follow-up for women whose cancer is in remission. However, these women are likely to need aftercare and support during recovery following primary treatment and should have continuing access to appropriate services. Care following primary treatment aims to identify and manage physical and psychological morbidity and to detect recurrent disease and initiate treatment as early as possible. Women should be informed about specific problems that may develop some time after treatment.

Organisation and provision of services

The optimum management of endometrial cancers requires close coordination between the primary healthcare team, the treatment teams at the cancer unit and cancer centre, the palliative care team and patients and their families. Effective communication is essential between all care settings. Decisions about management should follow local clinical policy, which should be demonstrably evidence based. All members of teams should be involved in discussions on local policy decisions and auditing adherence to them. Teams should be jointly responsible for audit and participation in clinical trials.

For endometrial cancer, the cancer unit should provide a rapid and appropriate assessment service at the local level for women presenting with postmenopausal bleeding. The designated lead gynaecologist should normally carry out surgery for early (stage Ia or Ib, grade 1 or 2) cancers of the endometrium. Specialist support from a cancer centre should be available, if needed. Women with late-stage endometrial cancers should be referred to the cancer centre following initial assessment at the cancer unit, since these are relatively uncommon and may present particular challenges. It is crucial to have mutually agreed criteria for rapid referral and effective channels of communication between primary care, cancer units and cancer centres.

References

1. Gull B, Carlsson S, Karlsson B, Ylostalo P, Milsom I, Granberg S. Transvaginal ultrasonography of the endometrium in women with postmenopausal bleeding: is it always necessary to perform an endometrial biopsy? *Am J Obstet Gynecol* 2000;182:509–15.

2. Ferrazzi E, Torri V, Trio D, Zannoni E, Filiberto S, Dordoni D. Sonographic endometrial thickness: a useful test to predict atrophy in patients with postmenopausal bleeding. An Italian multicenter study. *Ultrasound Obstet Gynecol* 1996;7:315–21.

3. Stovall TG, Solomon SK, Ling FW. Endometrial sampling prior to hysterectomy. *Obstet Gynecol* 1989;73:405–9.

4. Dijkhuizen FP, Mol BW, Brolmann HA, Heintz AP. The accuracy of endometrial sampling in the diagnosis of patients with endometrial carcinoma and hyperplasia: a meta-analysis. *Cancer* 2000;89:1765–72.

5. Frei KA, Kinkel K, Bonel HM, Lu Y, Zaloudek C, Hricak H. Prediction of deep myometrial invasion in patients with endometrial cancer: clinical utility of contrast-enhanced MR imaging: a meta-analysis and Bayesian analysis. *Radiology* 2000;216:444–9.

6. Kinkel K, Kaji K, Yu KK, Segal MR, Lu Y, Powell CB, *et al.* Radiologic staging in patients with endometrial cancer: a meta-analysis. *Radiology* 1999;212:711–18.

7. Eltabbakh GH, Shamonki MI, Moody JM, Garafano LL. Laparoscopy as the primary modality for the treatment of women with endometrial carcinoma. *Cancer* 2001;15:378–87.

8. Creasman WT, Morrow CP, Mundy BN. Surgical pathological spread patterns of endometrial cancer: a Gynecologic Oncology Group Study. *Cancer* 1987;60:2035–41.

9. Creutzberg CL, van Putten WL, Koper PC, Lybeert ML, Jobsen JJ, Wárlám-Rodenhuis CC, *et al.* Surgery and postoperative radiotherapy versus surgery alone for patients with stage-1 endometrial carcinoma: multicentre randomised trial. PORTEC Study Group. Post Operative Radiation Therapy in Endometrial Carcinoma. *Lancet* 2000;355:1404–11.

10. Creutzberg CL, van Putten WL, Wárlám-Rodenhuis CC, van den Bergh AC, de Winter KA, Koper PC, *et al.* Outcome of high-risk stage IC, grade 3, compared with stage I endometrial carcinoma patients: the Postoperative Radiation Therapy in Endometrial Carcinoma Trial. *J Clin Oncol* 2004;22:1234–41.

11. Podratz K, Mariani A, Webb M. Staging and therapeutic value of lymphadenectomy in endometrial cancer. *Gynecol Oncol* 1998;70:163–4.

12 Mariani A, Webb MJ, Galli L. Potential therapeutic role of paraaortic lymphadenectomy in node positive endometrial cancer. *Gynecol Oncol* 2000;76:348–56.

13. Chan JK, Wu H, Cheung MK, Shin JY, Osann K, Kapp DS. The outcomes of 27,063 women with unstaged endometrioid uterine cancer. *Gynecol Oncol* 2007;106:282–8.

14. ASTEC study group. Kitchener H, Swart AM, Qian Q, Amos C, Parmar MK. Efficacy of systematic pelvic lymphadectomy in endometrial cancer (MRC ASTEC Trial): A randomised study. *Lancet* 2009;373:125–36.

15. Panici PB, Basile S, Maneschi F, Alberto Lissoni A, Signorelli M, Scambia G, *et al.* Systematic pelvic lymphadenectomy vs. no lymphadenec-tomy in early-stage endometrial carcinoma: randomized clinical trial. *J Natl Cancer Inst* 2008;100:1707–16.

16. Nunns D, Williamson K, Swaney L, Davey M. The morbidity of surgery and adjuvant radiotherapy in the management of endometrial carcinoma. *Int J Gynecol Cancer* 2000;10:233–8.

17. Johnson N, Cornes P. Survival and recurrent disease after postoperative radiotherapy for early endometrial cancer: systematic review and meta-analysis. BJOG 2007;14:1313–20.

18. Creutzberg CL, van Putten WL, Koper PC, Lybeert ML, Jobsen JJ, Warlam-Rodenhuis CC, *et al.* Surgery and postoperative radiotherapy versus surgery alone for patients with Stage I endometrial carcinoma: multicenter randomised trial. *Lancet* 2000;355:1404–11.

19. Martin-Hirsch PL, Lilford RJ, Jarvis GJ. Adjuvant progestagen therapy for the treatment of endometrial cancer: review and meta-analyses of published randomised controlled trials. *Eur J Obstet Gynecol Reprod Biol* 1996;65:201–7.

11 Cervical cancer standards of care

Introduction

Many of the downward changes in the mortality trend for cervical cancer described in Chapter 1 are attributable to behavioural trends and to the introduction of the NHS Cervical Screening Programme. Further reductions in incidence may be seen in future following the introduction of a national human papillomavirus vaccination programme for girls aged 12–13 years of age in September 2008. However, there are still approxi-mately 2900 new cases of cervical cancer a year, of whom about 1000 will die.[1] It is hoped that, by achieving high standards of care for those women diagnosed with cervical cancer, deaths may be further reduced but also that this will bring improvements in women's quality of life, irrespective of whether or not they are curable, at all stages of their treatment pathway.

Multidisciplinary team working

Cervical cancer is now an uncommon disease and may present many complex challenges to clinicians and health workers from a wide variety of clinical specialties. It is now accepted that it is therefore appropriate for all cases of cervical cancer to be managed within a gynaecological oncology multidisciplinary team to ensure the consistent provision of the highest standards of care.

CURRENT STANDARD

All women with a cervical cancer should be referred to a gynaecological oncology multidisciplinary team.

Presentation

Women with early-stage disease may or may not have symptoms. Women who are asymptomatic may be detected because of an abnormal appear-ance of the cervix during clinical examination. This should prompt urgent referral for gynaecological assessment within 2 weeks. Women may also present as a result of abnormal cervical cytology. While a cervical smear cannot diagnose an invasive process, as it is an investigation of cytological abnormality it can suggest this if highly atypical cells are seen. Even in those women where the cervical smear report is suggestive of a preinvasive lesion, there still remains the possibility that the lesion may be cancerous. Careful colposcopy will pick up many of these lesions and will allow appropriate biopsies to be taken for diagnosis.[2] Any woman who has a smear suggestive of invasion or of glandular neoplasia should be referred urgently for colposcopy within 2 weeks; those with high-grade cytological abnormality should be referred and seen at a colposcopy clinic within 4 weeks.

Women of all stages of disease may present with symptoms. The symptoms associated with cervical cancer are dependent on the stage of disease. They are symptoms that are also associated with benign disease and, hence, are common and non-specific. The most frequent symptoms include postcoital bleeding, intermenstrual bleeding, postmenopausal bleeding or persistent vaginal discharge. Postcoital bleeding in younger women has a low risk of underlying cancer and these women should be tested for *Chlamydia trachomatis* before considering gynaecological referral. Women presenting with symptoms of cervical cancer (postcoital bleeding in women over 40 years, intermenstrual bleeding and persistent vaginal discharge) should be referred for gynaecological examination and onward referral for colposcopy if cancer is suspected. It is essential to be aware that a recent negative cervical smear does not exclude malignancy, as a necrotic tumour may not desquamate abnormal cells. Similarly, an abnormality of the cervix that raises the suspicion of malignancy indicates referral for further investigation irrespective of the cervical smear report.

Comprehensive treatment guidelines and quality standards for cervical screening and the management of abnormal smears have been published by the Cervical Screening Programme (see Chapter 4).

CURRENT STANDARD

- A clinically suspicious cervix should prompt referral. A negative cervical smear does not exclude cancer.
- Smears suggestive of malignancy or glandular neoplasia should be referred for colposcopy within 2 weeks.
- Smears suggestive of high grade dysplasia should be referred for colposcopy within 4 weeks.

Diagnosis and staging

A woman presenting to her general practitioner with intermenstrual bleeding or persistent vaginal discharge, or whose cervix looks or feels abnormal, should be referred to a gynaecologist. If there is a high index of suspicion that a malignancy is present, she should be referred to the gynaecological assessment service at a cancer unit rather than to a general gynaecologist and obstetrician.

Diagnosis is based upon a biopsy. If the lesion is large and clinically highly suspicious, then a directed biopsy will often suffice. In smaller

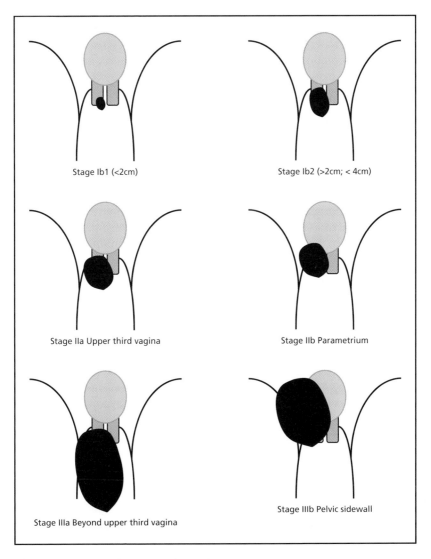

Stage Ib1 (<2cm)

Stage Ib2 (>2cm; < 4cm)

Stage IIa Upper third vagina

Stage IIb Parametrium

Stage IIIa Beyond upper third vagina

Stage IIIb Pelvic sidewall

Figure 11.1 Cervical staging schematic

lesions and especially in microscopic cancer (stage IA), the whole lesion should be included in the biopsy to allow for accurate histological sub-staging. This will most likely require either a cone biopsy or a large-loop or laser excision. If invasive disease is confirmed at histology a specialist pathologist at a cancer centre should also review the specimen in order to check the accuracy of staging. Histopathological reports should follow the minimum dataset of the Royal College of Pathologists.

The staging system for cervical cancer was reviewed by the FIGO in 2009.[3] Subsequent management depends on the stage of the disease (Figure 11.1; Appendix 1). If the specimen obtained at large-loop excision of the transformation zone (LLETZ) or cone biopsy shows no evidence of tumour at the margins and it falls within the measurement parameters of stage Ia disease, these cases may be managed at cancer unit level by the lead oncology gynaecologist. If clinical or histological examination at the unit level suggests a higher stage of disease, the woman should be referred to the specialist gynaecological team within a cancer centre.

STAGING

Following histological confirmation, investigations focus on staging and treatment planning. The staging of cervical cancer is clinical and must not be changed because of subsequent findings. The following examinations are permitted by FIGO to assign a clinical stage to carcinoma of the cervix (Figure 11.1):

- palpation, inspection and colposcopy of the cervix
- endocervical curettage, hysteroscopy, cystoscopy and proctoscopy
- intravenous urography
- X-ray examination of the lungs and skeleton.

Treatment planning in most centres in the UK often involves other imaging modalities such as computed tomography (CT) or magnetic resonance imaging (MRI) but these are not considered in allocating a FIGO stage. Where available, MRI scanning has been shown to be superior to clinical staging in assessing the extent of the disease.[1]

In women who undergo surgery, histopathological examination is used to assess the requirement for adjuvant therapy.

OTHER INVESTIGATIONS

It is essential that staging is performed in an accurate and systematic manner, to maximise the chances of a woman receiving the most appropriate management. In the UK, it is hoped that the development of cancer networks will lead to an improvement in the adequacy of staging, which previously has been shown to be less than ideal. An audit of cervical cancer during the 1989–93 period revealed that a large proportion of women were not correctly staged initially: 58% of women with higher than stage Ia disease had no X-ray performed preoperatively, 47% had no FIGO staging described in their notes and around 10% had inappropriate conservative surgery and subsequently required salvage surgery or radiotherapy.[4] It has also been shown that the type of hospital in which the staging is undertaken affects the staging adequacy. Teaching hospitals, with oncology support, have a higher adequacy of staging rate compared with non-teaching hospitals, without oncology support.[5] The obvious concern is that inadequate staging could lead to under-treatment, with potentially disastrous consequences, and conversely that over-staging could lead to unnecessary morbidity associated with therapy.

Although the disease is staged clinically, there is an increasing use of imaging techniques. The use of MRI scanning is now a standard part of the assessment process and has been shown to be superior to CT and clinical examination in terms of determining extent of tumour.[6,7] MRI has now replaced the intravenous urogram for assessment of hydroureter and hydronephrosis and is also the optimal test for determining lymph node status when compared with CT and lymphangiography.[8] The MRI should ideally be performed before any large biopsies, since the presence of inflammation may make interpretation of the scans more difficult and less reliable. If there are contraindications to MRI then CT is appropriate.

The role of positron emission tomography in scanning is currently under evaluation but it may offer superior detection of nodal metastasis. The use of a routine chest X-ray to exclude pulmonary metastases is appropriate for those with stage IIB disease or higher, where it has been shown to detect metastases in 4% of women.[9] However, it may not be justified for those with stage IB disease where there is a very low likelihood of pulmonary metastases.

CURRENT STANDARD

- Large biopsies including the whole lesion are required to accurately substage stage Ia disease.
- Pathological review of invasive disease should be undertaken by a specialist pathologist at a cancer centre and reports should follow the minimum dataset of the Royal College of Pathologists.
- Stage Ia disease can be managed in cancer units.
- Accurate staging is an essential prerequisite to good treatment planning.
- MRI is the radiological investigation of choice as an adjunct to clinical staging.

Treatment of cervical cancer

STAGE IA

Surgery is appropriate for the majority of women with stage IA cervical cancer (see also Chapter 5). For very early disease (stage IA1, where the depth of invasion is less than 3 mm) the incidence of positive lymph nodes is around 1% (negligible if less than 1 mm) and so, for the majority of women, local excision with LLETZ or cone biopsy is likely to be sufficient. In selected cases where there is lymphovascular space invasion (LVSI) consideration may be given to pelvic lymphadenectomy. Obviously, this decision has to be made with the informed consent of the patient.

When the depth of invasion is 3–5 mm, the risk of positive lymph nodes increases to around 4%. The incidence of node positivity in stage IA2 disease has been variably reported and lymphadenectomy should be considered, particularly in those who show evidence of LVSI and those with tumour volumes greater than 500 mm.[3,10,11] In cases of stage IA disease, local excision is usually sufficient to achieve local control. Thus, fertility can be spared in those women who wish to retain it. There is no evidence to support the use of radical surgery in stage IA disease.

Current standard

- Local excision is sufficient treatment for stage IA1 disease.
- Stage IA2 disease can also be managed by local excision but consideration of pelvic lymphadenectomy should be carried out on an individual case basis.
- Fertility sparing is possible in all stage IA disease.
- As parametrial involvement is not reported in stage-Ia disease, radical surgery is not necessary.

STAGE IB AND IIA

The currently available evidence would suggest that surgery (see also Chapters 5 and 6) and radiotherapy (see also Chapter 7) are equally effective in the treatment of stage IB cervical cancer. It is possible, although as yet not proven, that chemoradiation may offer improved outcomes. Surgery and radiotherapy have different morbidity profiles that will usually have the major influence on decision making. As with stage IA disease, women with small stage IB tumours (usually stage IB1) may have scope to retain their fertility. This group of women may be offered treatment by lymphadenectomy with trachelectomy, a procedure that has been reported to result in successful pregnancies.[12,13] Higher pregnancy rates and reduced complication rates might be offered by replacing radical trachelectomy with cervical cone biopsy in highly selected cases of small-volume disease with no adverse prognostic features. This is a crucial area for decision making by the woman and her partner and should only be undertaken after close liaison with the gynaecological oncology team in the cancer centre setting.

For women who do not wish to retain their fertility and for whom local excision would be an inadequate surgical treatment, the choice lies between radical hysterectomy with pelvic lymphadenectomy or radical radiotherapy. Both are equally effective in terms of outcome. Radical surgery should be carried out by specialist gynaecological oncologists working in cancer centres. It has been shown that radicalism of surgery is appropriately greater when patients are treated in specialist centres and that the 5-year survival of these women is increased.[5,14] Surgery alone should be offered whenever possible, since it is less likely to result in impaired sexual enjoyment, bowel or bladder function. If the woman is not fit to undergo surgery or she elects to be treated by radiotherapy, she should be offered radiotherapy. Most centres would now consider chemoradiation as the optimal form of treatment. For early-stage cervical disease, this has been shown to be as effective in terms of survival.[15–18]

Radiotherapy carries the risk of radiation-associated morbidity, including diarrhoea, cystitis and tiredness during or soon after the treatment and an 8% risk of long-term adverse affects, including problems with the bladder, bowel and vagina. Pelvic radiotherapy in younger women may also precipitate menopause and lead to infertility.

Adjuvant radiotherapy is widely used after radical surgery to reduce the risk of recurrence in women with positive nodes. Although it has been shown in several retrospective studies that adjuvant radiotherapy reduces the risk of recurrences within the pelvis, there is no firm evidence that it increases long-term survival.[18,19] Radical radiotherapy should be offered when surgery is unlikely to remove the tumour completely or when the risk of requiring postoperative radiation is considered high. This will help to reduce the number of cases where surgery and radiotherapy are employed as this has been shown to be associated with even higher levels of morbidity. A clinical oncologist with a specialist interest in gynaecological oncology should administer radiotherapy and chemoradiation. This is usually given in the form of intracavitary brachytherapy and external beam radiotherapy. The question of whether to give extended field radiotherapy (beyond the pelvic nodes) has been addressed in a number of studies.[20,21] Overall, there does not seem to be a significant benefit from extended field irradiation for all cases, as there is a significant increase in radiotherapy-related morbidity. However, it may prove to be appropriate in cases of proven para-aortic node involvement.

Current standard

- Surgery and radiotherapy are equally effective in terms of survival. Choice of therapy will depend on morbidity and patient choice.
- Radical trachelectomy with lymphadenectomy allows scope for fertility sparing in some women who have small (stage IB1) tumours.
- Members of the multidisciplinary team who have special expertise in the disease should give radical surgery and radiotherapy in gynaecological cancer centres.
- No benefit has been demonstrated from the use of extended field radiation.

LOCALLY ADVANCED (STAGE IIB AND ABOVE)

These cases do not usually lend themselves to primary surgical management. Treatment is based on radiotherapy and chemotherapy. A significant development in the management of cervical cancer has occurred in the last 3 years. Several randomised controlled trials have shown that concurrent platinum-based chemotherapy given with radiotherapy significantly improves survival and progression-free survival among women with disease ranging from stage IB–IVA when compared with the use of radiotherapy without chemotherapy.[22–25] The majority of centres in the UK now use a regimen of chemoradiation for these patients. An increasing number of these centres are also using chemotherapy for those women receiving adjuvant radiotherapy where nodal disease is present in women who have undergone radical surgery. While the results of these studies showed the efficacy of cisplatin in this setting, there is a gradual move towards the use of carboplatin in the UK.

Current standard

- Primary management is based on radiotherapy.
- Chemoradiation may be superior to radiotherapy alone, albeit with higher morbidity.
- Radiation with concurrent platinum is the combination of choice.

EXENTERATIVE SURGERY

For those women with extensive cancer confined to the central pelvis (recurrent cancer of the cervix or extensive primary disease), exenterative surgery can be considered if the woman is suitably fit and understands the risks and likely outcomes associated with such extensive surgery. Where the patients are carefully selected and the surgery is performed by highly skilled surgeons, a 5-year survival rate of 40–60% has been reported.[26–28] The surgical morbidity associated with this surgery is around 2–4%. In the three reporting studies above, a common finding was a zero percent survival rate (1–5 years) in those women found to be node-positive. This level of surgery should only be undertaken in cancer centres and only by those surgeons who are performing this type of surgery on a regular basis. In the future this may require the development of supra-regional centres. It is essential that careful preoperative counselling is given to these women, as they will have to undergo diversion of the urinary and/or gastrointestinal tracts and this is likely to have a major impact on their psychological, social and sexual function. Patients should then receive counselling from an appropriately trained and informed member of the multidisciplinary oncology team, typically the consultant performing the surgery and one of the nurse specialists from the team.

Current standard

- Exenterative surgery is highly specialized and should be performed only by expert teams in cancer centres.
- Women with positive lymph nodes do not benefit from this type of surgery.
- Patients should be carefully counselled with regard to the risks and morbidity of this type of surgery.

Post-treatment support and follow-up

There is no reliable evidence on which to base recommendations for routine follow-up of women who are asymptomatic after treatment for cervical cancer. In the majority of cancer centres in the UK, patients are followed up for 5 years and then discharged if all is well. No evidence supports the use of cervical cytology in follow-up and this practice should be discouraged.

There is one possible role for cytology in follow up. This is when there is a high index of suspicion of residual vaginal intraepithelial neoplasia. For this reason, all women undergoing surgery for cervical cancer should first have the vaginal vault assessed colposcopically to determine if the atypical transformation zone involves the vagina.

Treatment for all gynaecological cancers can result in physical, psychosocial and sexual morbidity. In the immediate postoperative period, the woman should, through local policy, receive help, support and appropriate treatment without delay, if it is required. They should be informed of specific problems that may develop some time after treatment for cervical cancer, such as lymphoedema, bowel or bladder dysfunction, and should have clear routes for access to appropriate specialist help if signs or symptoms appear. This will depend upon close liaison between cancer centres and units, general practitioners and supporting nursing care. These are principles that apply to all the gynaecological cancers.

When ovarian function is lost, as a result of either surgery or radiotherapy for cervical cancer, hormone replacement therapy should be considered. This treatment will relieve menopausal symptoms and has also been shown to be effective in reducing long-term rectal, bladder and vaginal complications of radiotherapy.[29]

CURRENT STANDARD

- Although there are no data to support the regular use of routine follow-up in treated patients, it may be of value in the early detection of recurrence, late morbidity and in providing psychological support for patients.
- The routine use of cervical cytology should be restricted to those in whom there is a high degree of suspicion that they may develop vaginal intraepithelial neoplasia.

Management of recurrent disease

One of the objectives of follow-up is to detect recurrent disease. Although many believe that the early detection of recurrence will positively influence the outcome of subsequent therapy, no data exist to support this.

Disease may relapse centrally, in the pelvis, at the pelvic side wall or by widespread and distant metastases. Adjuvant radiation is often given after primary surgery to reduce the risk of central pelvic relapse. If patients have received primary radiotherapy as their sole treatment, detecting pelvic relapse may be difficult, as it is not always easy to distinguish post-radiation fibrosis from recurrence. If doubt persists after imaging, Trucut® biopsies may be required to confirm recurrence.

CENTRAL PELVIC RELAPSE

Central pelvic relapse may present with dull central pelvic pain, bleeding or discharge. There may be alterations in either bowel or bladder function. The condition may be asymptomatic. If the central pelvic disease remains mobile, exenteration may be a treatment option. If the disease is fixed and the woman has not been treated previously by radiotherapy, this would be the first choice of treatment. Most centres would probably consider chemoradiation if the woman were fit, although none of the published data on chemoradiation specifically addresses the issue of relapsed disease.

PELVIC SIDE WALL RECURRENCE

The symptoms associated with recurrence on the side wall may relate to nerve root involvement (groin and leg pain), lymphatic occlusion (lymph-oedema in the affected limb), ureteric compression (usually asymptomatic) or visceral pain. A fixed mass palpable on the side wall in association with confirmatory imaging is usually considered diagnostic, although Trucut® or image-guided biopsies may be required. These cases are not amenable to further surgery and definitive treatment is by radiation, if not previously treated. In previously irradiated patients, treatment will usually be palliative in the form of pain control and/or chemotherapy. The results of chemotherapy are disappointing in previously irradiated tumours although a small improvement in median survival has been demonstrated with the use of a combination of cisplatin and topotecan.[30]

CURRENT STANDARD

- Mobile central pelvic recurrence can be managed by pelvic exenteration in selected patients.
- In previously non-irradiated women, central pelvic and side wall recurrence should be managed by radiotherapy.
- Although chemoradiation is considered in relapsed disease, no data are as yet available to show that this is superior to radiotherapy alone.
- Bone metastases are best managed by radiotherapy.
- Chemotherapy may have a role in the treatment of soft-tissue metastases that are not in previously irradiated sites.

DISTANT METASTASES

The presentation of distant metastases varies with the site and type of metastasis. Bone metastases will usually present with pain and can be well controlled by radiotherapy. Soft-tissue metastases will usually be considered for chemotherapy and reasonable response rates have been recorded in previously non-irradiated tissues. There are few long-term survivors in women with recurrent carcinoma of the cervix.

References

1. Cancer Research UK. Latest UK Cancer Incidence and Mortality Summary – numbers. July 2009 [http://publications.cancerresearchuk.org/WebRoot/cruk storedb/CRUK_PDFs/mortality/IncidenceMortalitySummary.pdf].
2. Shafi MI. Cervical cancer. In: Shafi MI, Luesley DM, Jordan JA, editors. *Handbook of Gynaecological Oncology*. London: Churchill Livingstone; 2000.
3. Pecorrelli S. Revised FIGO staging for carcinoma of the vulva, cervix and endometrium. *Int J Gynecol Obstet* 2009;105:103–4.
4. Jackson S, Murdoch J, Howe K, Bedford C, Sanders T, Prentice A. The management of cervical carcinoma within the south west region of England. *Br J Obstet Gynaecol* 1997;104:140–44.

5. Wolfe CD, Tilling K, Bourne HM, Raju KS. Variations in the screening history and appropriateness of management of cervical cancer in South East England. *Eur J Cancer* 1996;32A:1198–204.

6. Bipat S, Glas AS, van der Velden J, Zwinderman AH, Bossuyt PM, Stoker J. Computed tomography and magnetic resonance imaging in staging of uterine cervical carcinoma: a systematic review. *Gynecol Oncol* 2003;91:59–66.

7. Hricak H, Gatsonis C, Chi DS, Amendola MA, Brandt K, Schwartz LH, *et al*. Role of imaging in pretreatment evaluation of early invasive cervical cancer: results of the intergroup study American College of Radiology Imaging Network 6651–Gynecologic Oncology Group 183. *J Clin Oncol* 2005;23:29–37.

8. Scheidler J, Hricak H, Yu KK, Subak L, Segal MR. Radiological evaluation of lymph node metastases in patients with cervical cancer. A meta-analysis. *JAMA* 1997;278:1096–101.

9. Massad LS, Calvello C, Gilkey SH, Abu-Rustum NR. Assessing disease extent in women with bulky or clinically evident metastatic cervical cancer: yield of pre-treatment studies. *Gynecol Oncol* 2000;76:383–7.

10. Smith HO, Qualls CR, Romero AA, Webb JC, Dorin MH, Padilla LA, *et al*. Is there a difference in survival for 1A1 and 1A2 adenocarcinoma of the uterine cervix? *Gynecol Oncol* 2002;85:229–41.

11. Hirai Y, Takeshima N, Tate S, Akiyama F, Furuta R, Hasumi K. Early invasive adenocarcinoma: its potential for nodal metastasis or recurrence. *BJOG* 2003;110:241–6.

12. Shepherd JH, Crawford RAF, Oram DH. Radical trachelectomy: a way to preserve fertility in the treatment of early cervical cancer. *Br J Obstet Gynaecol* 1998;105:912–16.

13. Shepherd JH, Spencer C, Herod J, Ind TE. Radical vaginal trachelectomy as a fertility-sparing procedure in women with early-stage cervical cancer – cumulative pregnancy rate in a series of 123 women. *BJOG* 2006;113:719–24.

14. Bissett D, Lamont DW, Nwabineli NJ, Brodie MM, Symonds RP. The treatment of stage 1 carcinoma of the cervix in the west of Scotland 1980–1987. *Br J Obstet Gynaecol* 1994;101:615–20.

15. Landoni F, Maneo A, Colombo A, Placa F, Milani R, Perego P, *et al*. Randomised study of radical surgery versus radiotherapy for stage Ib–IIa cervical cancer. *Lancet* 1997;350:535–40.

16. Morley GW, Seski JC. Radical pelvic surgery versus radiation therapy for stage I carcinoma of the cervix (exclusive of microinvasion). *Am J Obstet Gynecol* 1976;126:785–98.

17. Newton M. Radical hysterectomy or radiotherapy for stage I cervical cancer. A prospective comparison with 5 and 10 year follow-up. *Am J Obstet Gynecol* 1975;123:535–42.

18. Soisson AP, Soper JT, Clarke-Pearson P, Berchuck A, Montana G, Creasman WT. Adjuvant radiotherapy following radical hysterectomy for patients with stage Ib and IIa cervical cancer. *Gynecol Oncol* 1990;37:390–5.

19. Kinney WK, Alvarez RD, Reid GC, Schray MF, Soong SJ, Morley GW, *et al*. Value of adjuvant whole pelvis irradiation after Wertheim hysterectomy for early stage squamous carcinoma of the cervix with pelvic nodal metastasis: a matched-control study. *Gynecol Oncol* 1989;34:258–62.

20. Rotman M, Pajak TF, Choi K, Clery M, Marcial V, Grigsby PW, *et al*. Prophylactic extended-field irradiation of para-aortic lymph-nodes in stage IIb and bulky Ib and IIa cervical carcinomas. Ten-year treatment results of RTOG 79-20. *JAMA* 1995;274:387–93.

21. Haie C, Pejovic MH, Gerbaulet A, Horiot JC, Pourquier H, Delouche J, *et al*. Is prophylactic para-aortic irradiation worthwhile in the treatment of advanced cervical cancer? Results of a controlled clinical trial of the EORTC radiotherapy group. *Radiother Oncol* 1998;11:101–2.

22. Rose PG, Bundy BN, Watkins EB, Thigpen JT, Deppe G, Maiman MA, *et al*. Concurrent cisplatin-based radiotherapy and chemotherapy for locally advanced cervical cancer. *N Engl J Med* 1999;340:1144–53.

23. Keys HM, Bundy BN, Stehman FB, Muderspach LI, Chafe WE, Suggs CL 3rd, *et al*. Cisplatin, radiation and adjuvant hysterectomy compared with radiation and adjuvant hysterectomy for bulky stage Ib cervical carcinoma. *N Engl J Med* 1999;340:1154–61.

24. Morris M, Eifel PJ, Lu J, Grigsby PW, Levenback C, Stevens RE, *et al*. Pelvic radiation with concurrent chemotherapy compared with pelvic and para-aortic radiation for high-risk cervical cancer. *N Engl J Med* 1999;340:1137–43.

25. Whitney CW, Sause W, Bundy BN, Malfetano JH, Hannigan EV, Fowler WC Jr, *et al*. Randomized comparison of fluorouracil plus cisplatin versus hydroxyurea as an adjunct to radiation therapy in stages IIb–IVa carcinoma of the cervix with negative para-aortic lymph nodes: a Gynecologic Oncology Group and Southwest Oncology Study Group. *J Clin Oncol* 1999;17:1339–48.

26. Robertson G, Lopes A, Beynon G, Malfetano JH, Hannigan EV, Fowler WC Jr, *et al*. Pelvic exenteration: a review of the Gateshead experience 1974–92. *Br J Obstet Gynaecol* 1994;101:529–31.

27. Shepherd JH, Ngan HS, Neven P, Fryatt I, Woodhouse CR, Hendry WF, *et al*. Multivariate analysis of factors affecting survival in pelvic exenteration. *Int J Gynecol Cancer* 1994;4:361–70.

28. Morley GW, Hopkins MP, Lindenauer SM, Roberts JA. Pelvic exenteration, University of Michigan: 100 patients at 5 years. *Obstet Gynecol* 1989;73:934–43.

29. Ploch E. Hormone replacement therapy in patients after cervical cancer treatment. *Gynecol Oncol* 1987;26:169–77.

30. Long HJ 3rd, Bundy BN, Grendys EC Jr, Benda JA, McMeekin DS, Sorosky J, *et al*. Randomised phase III trial of Cisplatin with or without topotecan in carcinoma of the uterine cervix: a Gynecologic Oncology Group study. *J Clin Oncol* 2005;23:4626–33.

12 Vulval cancer standards of care

Introduction

The rarity of vulval cancer has meant that few, if any, robust randomised trials have been performed. Evidence is based largely on personal series and is therefore subject to selection bias. Centralisation of care should have gone some way to allow properly designed trials to be conducted and there are data that also suggest that this may result in an improved outcome.[1–3]

CURRENT STANDARDS

- Vulval cancer should be managed in cancer centres by multidisciplinary teams.
- When considering standards of care in any disease situation, one of the primary areas to address is prevention: whether there is a preventative strategy that can be subjected to a quality assurance regimen.

Prevention and predisposing conditions

There is no screening strategy to either prevent invasive cancer of the vulva or to detect it at an early and asymptomatic stage. In approximately one-third of cases there will be evidence of a pre-existing human papillomavirus (HPV)-related disorder (vulval intraepithelial neoplasia, VIN)[4,5] and an additional one-third may have evidence of a vulval maturation disorder (such as lichen sclerosus). The aetiology is far from clear, however, and it is likely that there is more than one putative oncogenic process (see Chapter 1).

Women with Paget's disease of the vulva are not only at higher risk of having occult invasion at the time of diagnosis but may also be at higher risk than women with VIN of developing cancer in the future.[6] Melanoma in situ is also thought to be associated with a higher risk.[7,8]

An important point is that of follow-up in these at-risk conditions. It would seem impractical to offer regular follow-up to all women with a condition as common as lichen sclerosus, even though there is a roughly 4% lifetime risk of developing cancer.[9] Low-grade VIN is associated with a very low rate of progression to cancer and may not warrant follow-up. Current practice is to keep high-grade VIN, Paget's disease and melanoma in situ on annual review. Other predisposing conditions are assessed in a dedicated vulva clinic (preferably with multidisciplinary input). They may then be discharged from follow-up after counselling regarding level of risk and the changes in signs and symptoms that accompany malignant transformation. Their primary carers are also given this information and asked to review the women annually, with referral back to the vulva clinic as required.

CURRENT STANDARD

- There is no screening test for vulval cancer.
- Women with predisposing conditions should be counselled with regard to risk.
- Where risk is considered to be high, review should be arranged.

Referral from primary care

The incidence of vulval cancer is approximately 0.03 cases per 2000 population. Thus, in 10 years, the average general practitioner will see three cases. This rarity, combined with the modesty that women might feel owing to the intimate location of the problem means that a cancer might be easily overlooked, misdiagnosed or ignored. Simple accurate guidance for primary carers is therefore essential.

Although the disease can be asymptomatic, pain, itching, burning and soreness are the most frequent symptoms and almost 90% of women will admit to some symptoms. All symptomatic postmenopausal women and all premenopausal women not responding to simple first-line therapy should be examined. Genital warts are common but less so in the elderly and their presence should prompt early biopsy if not responding to simple topical therapies. Other features to look for include:

- a swelling, polyp or lump
- ulceration
- colour changes (whitening, loss or gain of pigment)
- elevation and/or irregularity of surface contour
- a clinical 'wart'
- irregular fungating mass
- ulcer with raised, rolled edges
- enlarged groin nodes.

Ninety percent of all vulval cancers will have an easily visible lesion at the time of first presentation.

CURRENT STANDARD

- All women with vulval symptoms should have the vulva examined.
- Any area of suspicious epithelium should prompt a gynaecological referral.
- Warts not responding to primary therapy should be biopsied.

Making the diagnosis

Diagnosis of vulval cancer is based on biopsy. Several scenarios may present themselves:

- a large fungating or ulcerated mass which is clinically malignant
- a small, well circumscribed mass that is suspicious for malignancy
- a lesion that has been biopsied is unexpectedly found to be cancerous.

FUNGATING OR ULCERATED MASS

A large fungating or ulcerated mass which is clinically malignant is unlikely to be resectable without significant morbidity and should therefore be biopsied from the edge of the lesion, so that adjacent normal looking epithelium is included in the specimen (Figure 12.1). This can occur under local anaesthesia, thus avoiding the risks of general

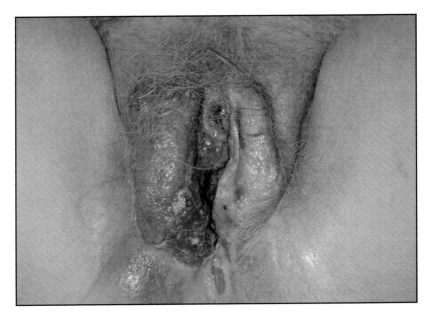

Figure 12.1 Diagnostic wedge biopsy should be taken from this tumour

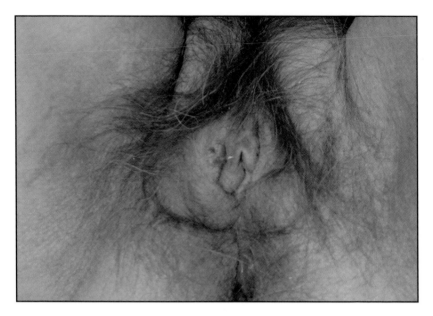

Figure 12.2 Excision biopsy of a small vulval lesion such as this is possible with margins of greater than 1cm in all planes

anaesthesia in women who are frequently elderly and frail. No attempt should be made to resect the lesion at this point.

SMALL, WELL CIRCUMSCRIBED MASS

Wide local excision with an adequate minimum resection margin of at least 1 cm (both deep and laterally) is frequently possible with minimal morbidity or functional deficit. It may be wise, however, still to perform a small biopsy, as in the first scenario (Figure 12.2). This is because subsequent sentinel node sampling is more difficult and potentially less reliable if there is no tumour present around which to inject the dye and radioisotope.

If primary wide local excision is undertaken, it is very important that adequate clearance margins are secured and that the site and size of the lesion are clearly recorded, using photography and the pathological records.

A LESION UNEXPECTEDLY FOUND TO BE CANCEROUS

Unless the malignancy is only microinvasive, re-excision will be a necessary part of subsequent treatment. Systems should be in place to ensure that unexpected cancers are flagged up in a timely fashion, the woman informed sensitively and the relevant referrals to a cancer centre instituted.

Biopsy information

Reporting standards in oncology are now becoming standardised. This ensures consistency, reproducibility, comparability and minimises confusion. In vulval cancer, the histopathology report should include reference to the following:

- benign or malignant
- histological type and grade
- depth of invasion (measured from base of nearest dermal papilla)
- clearance margins
- associated epithelial abnormalities
- involvement of capillary-like spaces (lymphovascular space invasion).

HISTOLOGICAL SUBTYPES

Knowledge of the subtype is important, as it may influence the need to assess lymph node status. Most squamous cancers of the vulva require assessment of nodal status. The only exceptions are verrucous and basal-cell carcinomas and squamous cancers with less than 1-mm depth of invasion (stage 1A). This superficially invasive disease carries less than 1% risk of nodal metastasis and the consensus is that nodal assessment is not required. Malignant melanoma is also considered a situation where lymph-adenectomy is not required, as long as there is no evidence of macro-scopically involved lymph nodes. The overwhelming prognostic determinant in this disease is depth of invasion (Clark's level) and not node status as it is in squamous disease. Prophylactic lymphadenec-tomy has not been shown to have independent prognostic or therapeutic significance in melanoma although some authorities feel that resection of bulky involved nodes may influence the course of the disease and at least confer some palliative benefit.

Current standard

- Diagnosis is based on a representative biopsy or biopsies from the most atypical areas.
- Diagnostic biopsies should include normal adjacent epithelium.
- Primary wide, local excision of small lesions may prejudice subsequent assessment of nodal status by sentinel node sampling and so, in centres where this is available, is best avoided.

Planning treatment

Once the diagnosis has been confirmed, treatment options need to be considered. The major factors that influence treatment planning are the need to assess nodal status, the extent of the disease and the woman's suitability for treatment. It may be necessary to consider additional investigations, such as imaging, to assess for bulky nodal disease and distant metastases. Other investigations to clarify comorbidity and suitability for treatment are undertaken at this point.

The importance of nodal status

Approximately 30% of all operated vulval cancers have involved lymph nodes and survival outcome correlates closely with lymph node status (Figure 12.3). The type of nodal involvement will also influence both outcome and choice of adjuvant therapy. Number and size of nodes involved and capsular breach are all pertinent[10,11] and the FIGO staging for vulval cancer was updated in 2009 to reflect this (see below).[12]

Nodal status has historically been determined by full dissection and clearance of superficial inguinal and deep femoral node bearing tissue, which then informs the decision on whether to use adjuvant radiotherapy. Groin dissection is a highly morbid procedure with significant rates, particularly of lymphoedema formation, but also of lymphocyst and wound breakdown. Missed and untreated groin disease, however, is highly symptomatic, is difficult to treat subsequently and carries a very poor prognosis. This has provided the justification for performing groin dissection in women

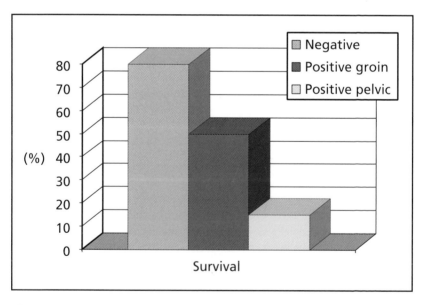

Figure 12.3 Survival in relation to nodal status

that we know have a less than one-third chance of deriving any benefit from the operation. Considerable effort has therefore been dedicated towards assessing nodal status by less invasive and morbid means.

The key factor of any putative nodal status assessment tool is that it should have virtually no false negatives. Imaging techniques such as computed tomography (CT), magnetic resonance imaging (MRI) and lymphangio-graphy have been used for this. Since they tend only to demonstrate macroscopic or bulky disease reliably, there is an unacceptably high false negative rate, accounted for by cases with small volume or microscopic nodal disease.

Another technique of nodal status assessment which has received widespread and growing attention is the use of sentinel node sampling.

SENTINEL NODE SAMPLING

Sentinel node sampling, already the standard of care in breast cancer and melanoma, is based on the concept that lymph channels serving a specific area of tissue (or tumour) will drain into an initial (or sentinel) locoregional lymph node. Any tumour spreading via this route, therefore, would be present in this node before then going on to spread sequentially to other nodes. If the sentinel nodes for a tumour can be reliably identified, sampled and found to be free of disease, it can be inferred that lymphatic metastasis has not yet occurred. This means the patient is spared full anatomical node dissection and the need for adjuvant treatment directed at nodal spread. Conversely, if the sentinel node is positive, this could trigger a full dissection to gain information about number of nodes involved. At the time of writing, the GROINSV-2 trial is in progress. This trial is evaluating simple recourse to adjuvant therapy for patients with positive sentinel nodes.[13]

In vulval cancer, the general consensus is that sentinel node identification should involve the combined use of blue dye and radioisotope injection. As the technique has developed, the following key points have been arrived at to minimise false negatives:

- The primary tumour should be no larger than 4 cm.
- If the primary tumour is central, sentinel nodes should be sought on both sides.
- Bulky nodal disease should have been excluded by CT, because a sentinel node replaced by tumour often fails to take up dye or radionucleotide.
- The technique has a distinct 'learning curve' and so should only be used without concomitant full groin dissection after at least ten procedures have been successfully carried out.
- Sentinel nodes sampled should be subjected to ultrastaging. This is a labour intensive and time-consuming method of histopathological

assessment which has been shown to demonstrate microscopic tumour deposits in the sentinel nodes of patients who have gone on to develop groin failure. Traditional haematoxylin and eosin staining and sectioning techniques are more likely to miss such cases.

- The technique should not be used if the primary tumour is multifocal.

By far the largest trial of sentinel node sampling in vulval cancer was the GROINSV-1 study in the Netherlands, which reported in 2008.[14] This study showed that, in 276 women with negative sentinel nodes, only eight had groin recurrence within 2 years (2.8%). This rate is comparable to that of the standard treatment of full groin dissection and confirms the safety of the technique relative to existing standards of care. It is important, however, to adhere scrupulously to the safety points described above,[15] as a trial in Germany which had more loosely defined criteria had a far higher false negative rate of 7.7%.[16]

Current standard

- Nodal status should be determined in all squamous cancers invading to a depth greater than 1 mm.
- This is usually achieved by unilateral or bilateral inguinofemoral node dissection, depending on tumour location.
- Nodal status may alternatively be assessed by sentinel node sampling, as long as the protocol for this is strictly adhered to.

Staging of vulval cancer

The FIGO system is used to describe the local, regional and distant extent of vulval cancer. It was updated in 2009 to reflect the complexities of nodal status and adjuvant therapy based on it (Table 12.1).[12]

Stage I disease is primarily managed by surgical excision.[17,18] This changes for disease more extensive than stage I. In these cases, where disease is not confined to the vulva but begins to involve adjacent structures or lymph nodes, there is a greater reliance on multidisciplinary treatment from the outset. An example of this might be to use radiotherapy or chemotherapy to reduce the volume (or occasionally eradicate disease) before surgery, in an attempt to minimise morbidity and preserve function. The same approach might be used for bulky nodes confirmed as positive, although there are few data on which to base this type of management. The stage of the disease is not the only variable considered when constructing a management plan. Other factors include:

- tumour size and depth
- tumour location in relation to other vital structures

Table 12.1 FIGO staging of carcinoma of the vulva

Stage	Description
I	Tumour confined to the vulva
Ia	Lesions ≤ 2cm in size, confined to the vulva or perineum and with stromal invasion ≤ 1 mm,[a] no nodal metastasis
Ib	Lesions > 2cm in size or with stromal invasion > 1 mm,[a] confined to the vulva or perineum, with negative nodes
II	Tumour of any size with extension to adjacent perineal structures (1/3 lower urethra, 1/3 lower vagina, anus) with negative nodes
III	Tumour of any size with or without extension to adjacent perineal structures (1/3 lower urethra, 1/3 lower vagina, anus) with positive inguinofemoral lymph nodes
IIIa	(i) with 1 lymph node metastasis (≥ 5mm) or (ii) 1–2 lymph node metatasis(es) < 5 mm
IIIb	(i) with 2 or more lymph node metastases (≥ 5mm) or (ii) 3 or more lymph node metatases < 5 mm
IIIc	With positive nodes with extracapsular spread
IV	Tumour invades other regional (2/3 upper urethra) or distant structures
IVa	Tumour invades any of the following: (i) upper urethral and/or vaginal mucosa, bladder mucosa, rectal mucosa or fixed to pelvic bone, or (ii) fixed or ulcerated inguinofemoral lymph nodes
IVb	Any distant metastasis, including pelvic lymph nodes

[a] The depth of invasion is defined as the measurement of the tumour from the epithelial–stromal junction of the adjacent most superficial dermal papilla to the deepest point of invasion

- tumour histology
- comorbidity
- patient wishes.

Managing the primary lesion

Historically, the standard of care for vulval cancer has been the performance of a radical vulvectomy with bilateral groin dissection via a single large butterfly-shaped incision. This is a morbid and disabling procedure. More recently, it has been demonstrated that wide local excision has a similar survival outcome at a lower morbidity cost, as long as a minimum clearance margin of 10 mm is achieved on all aspects of the tumour.[17,18] Adjacent atypical skin should be excised as well, although probably not to the same depth. Thus, small, localised tumours are adequately managed by wide local excision, while large multifocal lesions may still require complete removal of the vulva. Less morbidity also results if vulval surgery and groin surgery are performed through separate incisions.[19,20] This means that the butterfly incision has been consigned to history for the majority of women.

If adequate excision of the tumour will result in compromise of the urethra, anus or, in some instances, the clitoris, consideration should be given to prior downstaging treatment with radiation. There are some anecdotal data to support this approach by demonstrating that less radical and often sphincter-preserving procedures can accomplish adequate excision after radiotherapy.[21–22] Table 12.2 shows a summary of treatment options for different stages of disease.

Managing the lymph nodes

If the primary tumour is a basal-cell or verrucous carcinoma, or a malignant melanoma without suspicion of lymph node spread, then primary treatment does not require assessment of lymph node status. In all other cases, it does. Available evidence suggests that in unifocal stage I tumours which are lateralised, nodal assessment need only occur ipsilaterally through a separate incision from that treating the primary tumour. The incidence of disease in the contralateral groin is very low unless there is disease present in the ipsilateral groin. Thus, there is

Table 12.2 Treatment summary for vulval cancer		
Disease extent	*Description*	*Treatment principle*
Early	Stage IA	Wide local excision, no nodal assessment
	Lateralised IB	Wide local excision, ipsilateral groin dissection or sentinel node sampling
	Centralised IB	Wide local excision, bilateral groin dissection or bilateral sentinel node sampling
	Any IB > 4 cm	Adequate excision and groin dissection; no sentinel node sampling
Advanced	Stage II–IVA	Primary radiotherapy or radical surgery and bilateral groin dissection; no sentinel node sampling; plan tailored to patient
Metastatic	Stage IVB	Systemic chemotherapy and locoregional treatment with palliative intent (surgery and/or radiotherapy)

occasionally a need to perform a separate procedure for contralateral lymph node assessment. Central tumours mandate a bilateral lymph node assessment. A central tumour is defined as one which requires crossing of the midline to be adequately excised. Any tumour of the labium minus is also deemed to be central.

Data for choice of incision with bulky tumours and disease clinically involving lymph nodes are lacking. In these situations, there is potentially a higher risk of disease recurrence in the skin bridge between separate vulval and groin incisions. Use of the en bloc resection of vulva and groins via a single butterfly incision may thus still be indicated.

PELVIC NODES

Pelvic node involvement tends to follow inguinofemoral spread of disease. Previously, therefore, groin node involvement was a prompt to extend dissection to include iliac nodes in the pelvis. One randomised controlled trial, however, has suggested that women who have groin and pelvic irradiation after positive groin dissection fared better in terms of survival compared with those who had additional pelvic node dissection.[10] The difference, however, could be ascribed to improved groin disease control rather than any advantage experienced in the pelvis. One situation where pelvic node excision may prove beneficial is when there is bulky disease here, because radiotherapy in this instance has not proven to be particularly effective.

CURRENT STANDARDS

- Wide local excision is as effective as radical vulvectomy in early disease. All excision margins should be at least 10 mm.
- Preoperative radiotherapy should be considered if primary surgery is likely to compromise sphincter function.
- Large or multifocal lesions may still necessitate radical vulvectomy.
- Management of primary tumour and nodes should be decided on their own merits.

Adjuvant radiotherapy: early disease

In this situation, it is intended that surgery should be the sole therapeutic modality. Occasionally, however, findings on histopathological assessment of the surgical specimen increase the risk of local relapse sufficiently to justify further treatment. This takes the form of radiotherapy, 45–50 Gy given to a depth of at least 8 cm. Fields tend also to include the pelvic nodes. Both sides should be considered for treatment if the contralateral side does not have histological confirmation of negativity.

INADEQUATE EXCISION MARGIN

If any histopathologically reported excision margin is less than 8 mm, further intervention should be considered. The options are re-excision or local irradiation. The choice rests on the modality which is likely to have a lesser effect on subsequent function. The smaller margin of 8 mm compared with the 10 mm previously cited refers to the tissue shrinkage that is known to occur during fixation.

POSITIVE LYMPH NODES

Current convention is based on observational series only. This dictates that adjuvant radiation should be directed at the groin and pelvic nodes on the affected side if:[10,11]

- one node contains metastasis of 5 mm or greater
- one node demonstrates capsular breach
- more than one node has any degree of involvement.

This convention is currently being challenged by the introduction of sentinel node sampling. Usually, positive sentinel node sampling triggers full groin dissection. If this dissection meets the criteria for adjuvant treatment above, then the patient is subjected to the significantly enhanced morbidity of being exposed to two treatment modalities in the same site. The GROINSV-2 trial in the Netherlands is comparing this approach with one of direct recourse to adjuvant radiotherapy if sentinel node sampling is positive (even if only on ultrastaging), thereby sparing the patient full groin dissection.[13]

CURRENT STANDARD

- Any more than 5 mm involvement of a single node is an indication for adjuvant groin and pelvic irradiation.
- Primary tumour excision margins of less than 8 mm after fixation should prompt consideration of re-excision or local irradiation.

Advanced vulval cancer

Advanced disease includes all cases where primary excision would compromise sphincter function or where there is evidence of nodal spread or distant metastasis (stage II and beyond). Clinical assessment of nodal involvement is notoriously inaccurate and, unless enlarged nodes are obviously malignant (ulcerating or fungating; Figures 12.4, 12.5) histological confirmation should always be sought. This can be easily achieved by fine-needle aspiration. If histological confirmation cannot be achieved then the primary approach should be surgical.

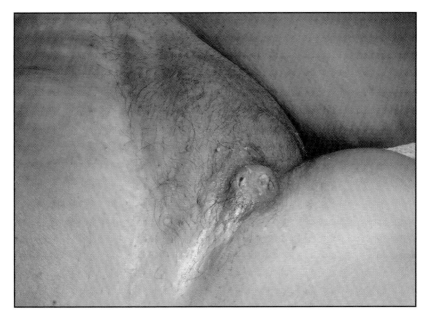

Figure 12.4 Fungating right groin node

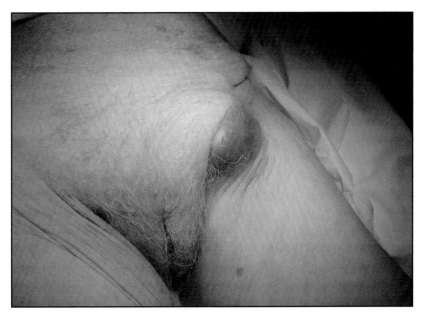

Figure 12.5 Enlarged malignant left groin node

MANAGEMENT OF GROSSLY INVOLVED NODES

There is no robust evidence to support either surgery or radiotherapy for primary treatment. If surgery is chosen as the primary modality, it will almost always be followed by adjuvant radiotherapy. The value of surgery following primary radiotherapy remains unclear. Hypothetically, initial surgery carries two advantages: necrotic bulk disease, which tends to be radioresistant, is removed before irradiation. Secondly, wound breakdown would appear less likely if surgery is performed on non-irradiated tissues.

COMBINED TREATMENT FOR THE PRIMARY

There have been several published series, albeit small, that would appear to support an approach of neoadjuvant radiotherapy in cases where the initial surgery would compromise sphincter function. These series are summarised in Table 12.3. They all appear to demonstrate that vulval cancer is sensitive to radiation, that tumour shrinkage does occur and that, in some at least, less compromising surgery can then be performed. In both the Hacker et al.[21] and Rotmensch et al.[22] series, patients were included if, at the outset, a colostomy would have been required to accomplish complete tumour clearance. Hacker avoided colostomy in all seven of his patients, with an overall survival rate of 62%, and Rotmensch avoided colostomy in 6 of 16, with overall survival of 45%. Whether these figures can be further improved with chemoradiation remains to be fully investigated. A Cochrane meta-analysis shows that neoadjuvant chemoradiation is effective but highly morbid and offers no information about effectiveness relative to radiation

Table 12.3 Published series supporting neoadjuvant radiotherapy in cases of vulval cancer where initial surgery would compromise function

Study	Cases (n)	Surgery	Residual tumour (%)	Survival (%)	Localised tumour (%)	Colostomy (n)
Acosta et al.[26]	14	RV+N	70	62	nk	2
Hacker et al.[21]	7	RLE+(N)	40	62	14	0
Boronow et al.[24]	37	RLE+(N)	57	76	14	4
Carson et al.[27]	8	RLE	25	25	nk	0
Rotmensch et al.[22]	16	RV+N	85	45	25	6
Wahlen et al.[28]	19	RLE	47	89	37	2
Lupi et al.[29]	24	RV+N	67	55	21	0

+N = and inguinofemoral nodes; RLE = radical local excision; RV = radical vulvectomy

given as a single modality.[23] The toxicity of single-modality vulval irradiation is considerable and likely to be greater with the addition of chemotherapy.

Some women will experience a complete response following radiotherapy. Whether surgery is necessary in such cases is also largely speculative. Current practice is to perform multiple biopsies from the tumour site 3 months following completion of surgery. Radical surgery is then deployed if residual disease is confirmed. If there has been a partial response, then radical excision with bilateral node dissection remains standard practice.

Reconstructive surgery

Reconstructive surgery may be required because of large tissue deficits that cannot be closed at the time of excision or because of a desire to retain as much function as possible, or for cosmetic reasons. The requirement for reconstruction should be considered in all patients undergoing surgery for vulval cancer.

A variety of rotational and transposition grafts have been used in vulval reconstruction and this depends on the site and size of the defect and the availability of suitable donor sites. Split skin may also be of value, particularly where the bulk of a transposition graft may not easily be accommodated or where there is a high risk of graft breakdown, such as in an infected site or when the patient is a heavy smoker.

The increasing use of reconstruction in vulval cancer management has made reconstructive surgeons an integral part of the multidisciplinary team. Gynaecological oncologists should, however, be trained in basic techniques, which will suffice in the majority of patients.

CURRENT STANDARD

- In locally advanced tumours, preoperative radiation or chemoradiation may reduce subsequent surgical morbidity
- Reconstruction should be considered and discussed in all cases where radical excision is contemplated.

Morbidity

Morbidity results as a consequence of:

- relapsed disease (local, regional, distant)
- structural or functional damage as a result of treatment
- psychosexual damage.

Either re-excision or radiation can manage local relapse and, generally, the modality less likely to result in functional deficit will be the first choice. In previously irradiated areas, the choice is usually limited to surgery. It is far preferable to try to avoid local recurrence by ensuring adequate excision margins during primary treatment. Reconstruction at the time of surgery is preferable if this allows wider margins and, while preservation of function is important, it should not compromise chance of cure.

Relapse in the groin is invariably incurable. Radiotherapy may be given if it has not been used before and excision has been attempted. The prognosis is poor and death from disease is highly likely. This underlines the importance of appropriate management planning at the outset.

POSTOPERATIVE MORBIDITY

The high morbidity and long hospital stay associated with radical vulvectomy have largely driven changes in care. While newer, more conservative approaches to treatment have improved morbidity, it is still seen more frequently and is more severe than one would wish. The major postoperative morbidities are:

- wound breakdown
- wound infection
- deep vein thrombosis and pulmonary embolism
- pressure sores.

Other morbidity becomes apparent at follow-up and this is one reason why follow-up is still considered important in this disease. Chronic problems that may arise include:

- introital stenosis
- incontinence (urinary and faecal)
- rectocele
- lymphocyst
- lymphoedema
- hernia
- psychosexual problems.

The introduction of sentinel node sampling has been shown to significantly reduce the risk of lymphoedema formation but did not appear to improve quality of life relative to standard treatment of full inguinofemoral node dissection.[24]

References

1. Penney GC, Kitchener HC, Templeton A. The management of carcinoma of the vulva: current opinion and current practice among consultant gynaecologists in Scotland. *Health Bull (Edinb)* 1995;53:47–54.

2. Rhodes CA, Cummins C, Shafi MI. The management of squamous cell vulval cancer: a population based retrospective study of 411 cases. *Br J Obstet Gynaecol* 1998;105:200–5.

3. van der Velden J, van Lindert AC, Gimbrere CH, Oosting H, Heintz AP. Epidemiologic data on vulvar cancer: comparison of hospital with population-based data. *Gynecol Oncol* 1996;62:379–83.

4. Jones RW, Baranyai J, Stables S. Trends in squamous cell carcinoma of the vulva: the influence of vulvar intraepithelial neoplasia. *Obstet Gynecol* 1997;90:448–52.

5. Herod JJ, Shafi MI, Rollason TP, Jordan JA, Luesley DM. Vulvar intraepithelial neoplasia: long term follow up of treated and untreated women. *Br J Obstet Gynaecol* 1996;103:446–52.

6. Fishman DA, Chambers SK, Schwartz PE, Kohorn EI, Chambers JT. Extramammary Paget's disease of the vulva. *Gynecol Oncol* 1995;56:266–70.

7. Ragnarsson-Olding B, Johansson H, Rutqvist LE, Ringborg U. Malignant melanoma of the vulva and vagina. Trends in incidence, age distribution, and long-term survival among 245 consecutive cases in Sweden 1960–1984. *Cancer* 1993;71:1893–7.

8. Bradgate MG, Rollason TP, McConkey CC, Powell J. Malignant melanoma of the vulva: a clinicopathological study of 50 women. *Br J Obstet Gynaecol* 1990;97:124–33.

9. Friedrich EG. Vulvar dystrophy. *Clin Obstet Gynecol* 1985;28:178–87.

10. Homesley HD, Bundy BN, Sedlis A, Adcock L. Radiation therapy versus pelvic node resection for carcinoma of the vulva with positive groin nodes. *Obstet Gynecol* 1986;68:733–40.

11. van der Velden J, van Lindert AC, Lammes FB, ten Kate FJ, Sie-Go DM, Oosting H, *et al.* Extracapsular growth of lymph node metastases in squamous cell carcinoma of the vulva. The impact on recurrence and survival. *Cancer* 1995;75:2885–90.

12. Pecorelli S. Revised FIGO staging for carcinoma of the vulva, cervix, and endometrium. *Int J Gynecol Obstet* 2009;105:103–4.

13. Groningen International Study on Sentinel Lymph Nodes in Vulvar Cancer II: an observational study, phase III [www.ikcnet.nl/trials/index.php?id=765] and [www.trialregister.nl/trialreg/admin/rctview.asp?TC=608].

14. Van der Zee AGJ, Oonk MH, De Hullu JA, Ansink AC, Vergote I, Verheijen RH, *et al.* Sentinel node dissection is safe in the treatment of early-stage vulvar cancer. *J Clin Oncol* 2008;26:884–9.

15. de Hullu JA, Oonk MHM, Ansink AC, Hollema H, Jager PL, van der Zee AGJ. Pitfalls in the sentinel lymph node procedure in vulvar cancer. *Gynecol Oncol* 2004;94:10–15.

16. Hampl M, Hantschmann P, Michels W, Hillemanns P. Validation of the accuracy of the sentinel lymph node procedure in patients with vulvar cancer: results of a multicenter study in Germany. *Gynecol Oncol* 2008;111:282–8.

17. Heaps JM, Fu YS, Montz FJ, Hacker NF, Berek JS. Surgical-pathologic variables predictive of local recurrence in squamous cell carcinoma of the vulva. *Gynecol Oncol* 1990;38:309–14.

18. Hacker NF, Van der Velden J. Conservative management of early vulvar cancer. *Cancer* 1993;71(4 Suppl):1673–7.

19. Stehman FB, Bundy BN, Dvoretsky PM, Creasman WT. Early stage I carcinoma of the vulva treated with ipsilateral superficial inguinal lymphadenectomy and modified radical hemivulvectomy: a prospective study of the Gynecologic Oncology Group. *Obstet Gynecol* 1992;79:490–7.

20. Hacker NF, Leuchter RS, Berek JS, Castaldo TW, Lagasse LD. Radical vulvectomy and bilateral inguinal lymphadenectomy through separate groin incisions. *Obstet Gynecol* 1981;58:574–9.

21. Hacker NF, Berek JS, Juillard GJ, Lagasse LD. Preoperative radiation therapy for locally advanced vulvar cancer. *Cancer* 1984;54:2056–61.

22. Rotmensch J, Rubin SJ, Sutton HG, Javaheri G, Halpern HJ, Schwartz JL, *et al.* Preoperative radiotherapy followed by radical vulvectomy with inguinal lymphadenectomy for advanced vulvar carcinomas. *Gynecol Oncol* 1990;36:181–4.

23. van Doorn HC, Ansink A, Verhaar-Langereis M, Stalpers L. Neoadjuvant chemoradiation for advanced primary vulvar cancer. *Cochrane Database Syst Rev* 2006;(3):CD003752.

24. Oonk MHM, van Os MA, de Bock GH, de Hullu JA, Ansink AC, van der Zee AGJ. A comparison of quality of life between vulvar cancer patients after sentinel lymph node procedure only and inguinofemoral lymphadenectomy. *Gynecol Oncol* 2009;113:301–5.

25. Boronow RC, Hickman BT, Reagan MT, Smith RA, Steadham RE. Combined therapy as an alternative to exenteration for locally advanced vulvovaginal cancer. II. Results, complications, and dosimetric and surgical considerations. *Am J Clin Oncol* 1987;10:171–81.

26. Acosta AA, Given FT, Frazier AB, Cordoba RB, Luminari A. Preoperative radiation therapy in the management of squamous cell carcinoma of the vulva: preliminary report. *Am J Obstet Gynecol* 1978;132:198–206.

27. Carson LF, Twiggs LB, Adcock LL, Prem KA, Potish RA. Multimodality therapy for advanced and recurrent vulvar squamous cell carcinoma. A pilot project. *J Reprod Med* 1990;35:1029–32.

28. Wahlen SA, Slater JD, Wagner RJ, Wang WA, Keeney ED, Hocko JM, *et al.* Concurrent radiation therapy and chemotherapy in the treatment of primary squamous cell carcinoma of the vulva. *Cancer* 1995;75:2289–94.

29. Lupi G, Raspagliesi F, Zucali R, Fontanelli R, Paladini D, Kenda R, *et al.* Combined preoperative chemoradiotherapy followed by radical surgery in locally advanced vulvar carcinoma. A pilot study. *Cancer* 1996;77:1472–8.

13 Uncommon gynaecological cancers

Introduction

The investigation and management of uncommon gynaecological cancers is based mainly upon cohort studies, case series and expert opinion. The evidence base is weak, with few randomised controlled trials available to guide the treatment of these tumours, due to their rarity. However, the management of gestational trophoblastic disease is more robust, as randomised controlled trials have been undertaken and treatment modified accordingly.

Gestational trophoblastic disease

Gestational trophoblastic disease (GTD) is defined as an excessive and inappropriate proliferation of the trophoblast. It includes a spectrum of disease from the benign hydatidiform mole (complete and partial), to the malignant gestational trophoblastic tumour (GTT): invasive mole, choriocarcinoma and the rare placental site trophoblastic tumour (PSTT).

Complete moles occur in about 1/1000 pregnancies and partial hydatidiform moles in 3/1000 pregnancies. Complete moles lack identifiable embryonic or fetal tissue and usually have a diploid 46XX karyotype, with entirely paternal chromosomes. Partial hydatidiform moles have identifiable embryonic or fetal tissue and usually have a triploid karyotype (69 chromosomes), with an extra haploid set of paternal chromosomes. The risk of developing malignant disease after suction evacuation of a complete mole is 15% (with metastases in 4%) and 2–4% after evacuation of a partial hydatidiform mole. The malignant tumour is usually an invasive mole but choriocarcinoma can arise in up to 3% of complete moles and, rarely, after a partial hydatidiform mole. Invasive moles invade the myometrium and are characterised by trophoblastic hyperplasia and the persistence of placental villous structures. In virtually all cases, they are preceded by a molar pregnancy and rarely progress to choriocarcinoma. They can metastasise to the lungs, vagina, brain, liver and, rarely, the skin, lymph nodes and bone. It does not progress like a true cancer and often regresses spontaneously. Choriocarcinoma arises from the trophoblast and contains both cytotrophoblast and syncytiotrophoblast. The lack of villous structures distinguishes it from an invasive mole. Choriocarcinoma can arise from any pregnancy, which may have occurred up to several years previously. More than 50% are preceded by a molar pregnancy and they are 1000 times more common after a complete mole than a normal pregnancy. They can metastasise.

Placental site trophoblastic tumour arises from the trophoblast of the placental bed and consists of mainly cytotrophoblastic cells, hence the relatively low level of human chorionic gonadotrophin (hCG) associated with this tumour. Human placental lactogen can be detected in both serum and immunohistochemically on histology. It is rare, with one case of PSTT for every 100 cases of invasive mole and choriocarcinoma. Treatment is by complete surgical excision as it is not a chemosensitive tumour.

FIGO STAGING OF GESTATIONAL TROPHOBLASTIC TUMOURS

In 1991, FIGO added nonsurgical pathologic prognostic risk factors to the anatomical staging system (Appendix 1). Risk factors affecting staging include urinary hCG levels greater than 100 000 miu/ml and/or serum hCG greater than 40 000 miu/ml and the duration of disease more than 6 months from termination of the antecedent pregnancy.

RISK FACTORS

Risk factors for GTD include:

- maternal age: teenagers have a slightly higher incidence than women aged 20–40 years and women over 40 years of age have a much higher incidence
- race: Asian women have higher rates of GTD than Arab and white women, with African American women having a low incidence
- reproductive history: women who have had a previous molar pregnancy are at much greater risk of another, compared with women who have never had a molar pregnancy
- parental blood groups: women with blood group A and whose partners are blood group O have a higher risk of choriocarcinoma
- genetic predisposition: familial clustering of GTD has been reported.

There are no environmental factors associated with GTD.

PRESENTATION AND DIAGNOSIS

Women with a partial hydatidiform mole usually present with the signs and symptoms of an incomplete or missed miscarriage. The diagnosis is often made on histology of the retained products of conception. Complete molar pregnancies present with signs and symptoms shown in Table 13.1. The diagnosis of a complete mole is now often made in the first trimester, either by the detection of raised hCG levels or by the classic vesicular 'snowstorm' ultrasound appearance.

INVESTIGATIONS

Preoperative investigations include:

- history and examination
- pelvic ultrasound scan
- full blood count/clotting, to exclude anaemia or clotting disorder
- urea and electrolytes, liver function tests, thyroid function tests, to exclude metastatic disease or hyperthyroidism
- crossmatch blood, as there is a risk of haemorrhage at evacuation.

Table 13.1 Signs and symptoms of complete molar pregnancy

Symptom	Occurrence (%)	Description
Vaginal bleeding		May cause anaemia; vesicles may also be passed vaginally
Excessive uterine size	≤ 50	Usually associated with very high levels of hCG, which may be > 200 000
Hyperemesis gravidarum		Due to the increased levels of hCG; may result in severe electrolyte disturbances
Toxaemia		Pre-eclampsia is also associated with an increased level of hCG; complete mole should be considered in any woman developing hypertension in the first trimester
Hyperthyroidism	c. 7	thought to be due to the thyrotropic activity of hCG
Trophoblastic embolisation	≤ 2%	Patients may have chest pain, tachypnoea, tachycardia and respiratory distress requiring cardiopulmonary support
Theca lutein ovarian cysts	≤ 50 (> 6 cm diameter)	Usually bilateral and multilocular and associated with markedly elevated serum hCG levels; normally regress spontaneously within 2–4 months, after evacuation

MANAGEMENT

Suction evacuation of the uterine cavity is the treatment of choice for molar pregnancy. This should be performed by an experienced surgeon, as there is an increased risk of perforation and haemorrhage. All tissue should be sent for histological examination.

After evacuation, patients should be registered with a UK supraregional centre (Charing Cross Hospital, London; Weston Park Hospital, Sheffield; or Ninewells Hospital, Dundee) and computerised hCG follow-up undertaken. Weekly serial hCG measurements should be taken until the level has returned to normal for 4 weeks. If the level reaches normal within 8 weeks of the diagnosis of molar pregnancy, follow-up is undertaken for 6 months, otherwise it is continued for 2 years. Patients should use effective contraception for 6 months following an evacuation for a molar pregnancy, to avoid confusion between a normal pregnancy and a rising hCG titre, indicating the development of invasive disease. Oral contraceptives can be used, as they do not increase the risk of post-molar trophoblastic disease.[1] hCG levels should be taken at 6 and 12 weeks post-delivery after any future pregnancy, owing to the increased risk of trophoblastic disease.

Approximately 8% of women registered in the UK with GTD will need adjuvant chemotherapy. The use of prophylactic chemotherapy in women who are unlikely to comply with follow-up is controversial. There is a theoretical risk that such women will develop drug resistance should they require chemotherapy for GTT in the future.

The World Health Organization Scientific Group agreed in 1983 that chemotherapy should be given to women who have had a partial hydatidiform mole when:

- a high level of hCG is present 4 weeks after evacuation: serum level greater than 20000 iu/l, urine level greater than 30000 iu/l (owing to the risk of uterine perforation)
- rising hCG levels at any time post-evacuation
- histological identification of choriocarcinoma or evidence of central nervous system, renal, hepatic or gastrointestinal metastases, or pulmonary metastases greater than 2 cm in diameter or more than three in number.

Charing Cross Hospital, London, will also give chemotherapy to women with persistent uterine haemorrhage or detectable hCG in serum or urine 4–6 months post-evacuation.

A number of prognostic variables have been identified and cases can be categorised into low-, medium- and high-risk,[2] so that patient treatment is stratified appropriately. This ranges from single-agent methotrexate plus folinic acid, etoposide or actinomycin D, to intensive drug combinations, such as EMA-CO (actinomycin D, etoposide, methotrexate, folinic acid, vincristine and cyclophosphamide). Charing Cross Hospital uses a modification of Bagshawe's prognostic scoring system.

Hysterectomy with adjuvant single-agent chemotherapy may be appropriate treatment for stage I GTD in women who do not wish to preserve fertility. It may also be required to control uterine haemorrhage or sepsis with metastatic GTT. In women with drug resistant disease, where the active site can be identified, salvage surgery is indicated. Success rates for salvage surgery are hysterectomy (15%), thoracotomy (43%) and craniotomy (71%).

FOLLOW-UP AND OUTCOME FOLLOWING CHEMOTHERAPY

After completion of chemotherapy, patients are followed up by serial serum and urine hCG estimations. Women are advised against pregnancy for a year after completing chemotherapy, to distinguish between a further pregnancy and relapsed disease. Women who have had a complete molar pregnancy can anticipate normal future reproductive function, with up to 77.5% having live births following chemotherapy. However, women who have had one molar pregnancy have a 1% risk of a further molar pregnancy.[3] Chemotherapy with etoposide may increase the rate of second tumours, such as acute myeloid leukaemia. The long-term survival of women treated for gestational trophoblastic tumour at Charing Cross Hospital is 94% at 15-year follow-up.

Cancer of the fallopian tube

Primary carcinoma of the fallopian tube is rare, accounting for 0.3% of all gynaecological malignancies. The majority of cancers are epithelial in origin, commonly serous but, rarely, sarcomas occur. Most tubal malignancies are secondary from the uterus, ovary, gastrointestinal tract or breast.

Tubal cancers occur most frequently in the fifth and sixth decades, with a mean age of 55–60 years. Many women with tubal cancer are nulliparous (45%) and many have a history of infertility.

FIGO STAGING OF CARCINOMA OF THE FALLOPIAN TUBE

Staging for fallopian tube carcinoma is by the surgical pathological system (Appendix 1). Operative findings prior to tumour debulking may be modified by histopathological, clinical or radiological evaluation.

PRESENTATION AND DIAGNOSIS

Primary adenocarcinoma of the fallopian tube can present with variable, non-specific symptoms:

- abdominal pain
- serosanguinous discharge (hydrops tubae profluens)
- pelvic mass
  (this triad of symptoms occurs in less than 15% of women)
- abnormal vaginal bleeding, often postmenopausal
- unexplained abnormal cervical cytology
- urinary or bowel disturbance.

Fallopian tube cancer is bilateral in 10–20% of cases and is often found incidentally in women who are asymptomatic, at the time of total abdominal hysterectomy and bilateral salpingo-oophorectomy (Figures 13.1, 13.2). Many present with early disease: 37% with stage I and 20% with stage II disease, respectively. Therefore, the overall 5-year survival rate for fallopian tube carcinoma is higher than that for epithelial ovarian cancer, which presents much later.

INVESTIGATIONS

Serum CA125 levels may be elevated in tubal carcinoma; CA125 titres may predict tumour presence and can monitor response to therapy. Routine preoperative tests required for any laparotomy for suspected gynaecological malignancy should be performed: full blood count, urea and electrolytes, liver function tests and chest X-ray. A pelvic/abdominal ultrasound scan should be performed. Computed tomography of the pelvis/abdomen may be useful to delineate tumour.

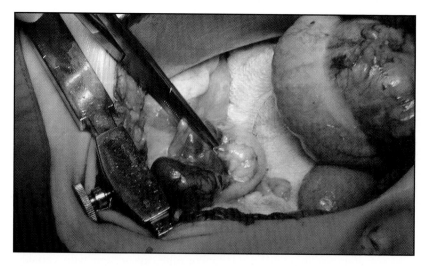

Figure 13.1 Left fallopian tube cancer

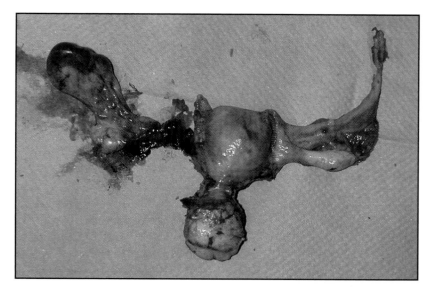

Figure 13.2 Hysterectomy specimen showing normal ovaries

MANAGEMENT

Laparotomy

The treatment of fallopian tube carcinoma is identical to that of epithelial ovarian carcinoma (see Chapter 9). Primary debulking surgery is performed to stage the disease and to attempt total macroscopic clearance. Unilateral salpingo-oophorectomy may be performed in young women with a stage IA well-differentiated tumour who are desirous of fertility.

Chemotherapy

Adjuvant cisplatin-based combination chemotherapy has been used in tubal carcinoma with up to an 80% response rate. Owing to the clinical and histological similarity between tubal and epithelial ovarian cancer, response rates and survival to chemotherapy are expected to be similar in the two groups. Currently, combination carboplatin and paclitaxel would be recommended (see also Chapter 8 Chemotherapy).

Radiation

Radiation therapy has frequently been used in the treatment of fallopian tube carcinoma in the past. However, the role of radiation in the management of this disease remains unclear. Whole-abdomen irradiation may improve survival in patients with completely resected disease or microscopic metastases[4] (see also Chapter 7 Radiotherapy).

Tubal sarcomas

Tubal sarcomas, mainly malignant mixed mesodermal tumours, are very rare. They usually present at an advanced stage in the sixth decade. Treatment is by primary debulking surgery and adjuvant combination chemotherapy. The overall 5-year survival rate for women with epithelial tubal carcinomas is 56%. The 5-year survival rates for women according to stage at presentation are 84% for stage I, 52% for stage II and 36% for stage III disease, respectively.

Nonepithelial ovarian cancers

Nonepithelial malignancies of the ovary account for approximately 10% of all ovarian cancers. They include germ-cell malignancies, sex-cord stromal tumours, metastatic carcinomas to the ovary and the rare lipoid cell tumours, sarcomas and small-cell carcinomas of the ovary.

OVARIAN GERM-CELL TUMOURS

Germ-cell tumours are derived from the primordial germ cells of the ovary. Although 20–30% of all ovarian neoplasms (both benign and malignant) are of germ cell origin, only approximately 3% are malignant. However, in the first two decades of life, almost 70% of ovarian tumours are of germ cell origin and one-third of these are malignant. Ovarian germ-cell tumours are

Class	Type
Table 13.2	**Histological typing of ovarian germ-cell tumours**
1	Dysgerminoma

2	Teratoma:
	    A. Immature
	    B. Mature: (1) Solid
	                  (2) Cystic a. Dermoid cyst (mature cystic teratoma)
	                                     b. Dermoid cyst with malignant transformation
	    C. Monodermal and highly specialised:
	                  (1) Struma ovarii
	                  (2) Carcinoid
	                  (3) Struma ovarii and carcinoid
	                  (4) Others

3	Endodermal sinus tumour
4	Embryonal carcinoma
5	Polyembryona
6	Choriocarcinoma
7	Mixed forms

staged as for epithelial ovarian carcinoma and are classified according to histological type (Table 13.2). Some ovarian germ-cell malignancies secrete hormones detectable in the serum: dysgerminomas secrete placental alkaline phosphatase and lactate dehydrogenase; endodermal sinus tumour secretes alphafetoprotein (AFP); embryonal carcinoma secretes AFP and hCG; choriocarcinoma secretes hCG.

Presentation and diagnosis

Germ cell malignancies grow rapidly and often present with pelvic pain, owing to capsular distension, haemorrhage or necrosis. The rapidly enlarging pelvic mass may cause bowel or bladder pressure symptoms or menstrual irregularities. Diagnosis can be delayed by a misdiagnosis of pregnancy. A germ-cell tumour should be suspected prior to surgery in a young woman with a predominately solid ovarian tumour; such women should be referred to a gynaecological oncologist.

Investigations

- Full blood count
- Urea and electrolytes
- Liver function tests
- Chest X-ray
- Pelvic/abdominal ultrasound scan
- CT scan pelvis/abdomen to exclude retroperitoneal lymphadenopathy and liver metastases
- hCG
- AFP
- Karyotype: premenarchal ovarian germ cell tumours often arise in dysgenetic gonads.

DYSGERMINOMAS

Dysgerminomas account for approximately 30–40% of all ovarian germ-cell tumours, representing only 1–3% of all ovarian cancers. However, they do account for 5–10% of ovarian cancers in women under 20 years of age, with 75% of dysgerminomas occurring between 10 and 30 years of age.[5] Approximately 5% are found in women with a female phenotype and abnormal gonads. Bilateral tumours are found in 10–15% and 75% of cases are stage I at presentation.

Management

Stage IA disease can be treated conservatively with unilateral salpingo-oophorectomy, providing appropriate staging has been undertaken to exclude occult metastatic disease. Advanced disease is treated by total abdominal hysterectomy and bilateral salpingo-oophorectomy and all women with a Y chromosome on karyotyping should have a bilateral oophorectomy.

Dysgerminomas are radiation-sensitive but chemotherapy has replaced radiotherapy to preserve fertility (see also Chapter 8 Chemotherapy). Advanced-stage or incompletely resected dysgerminomas are treated with four cycles of BEP (bleomycin, etoposide and cisplatin). In women with recurrent disease who have received prior BEP chemotherapy, POMB-ACE (cisplatin, vincristine, methotrexate, and bleomycin; and actinomycin D, cyclophosphamide and etoposide) may be used.

Outcome

Women with stage IA dysgerminomas treated by unilateral salpingo-oophorectomy have a 5-year survival rate greater than 95%. Combination chemotherapy now achieves cure rates of 90–100% for advanced disease.[6]

IMMATURE TERATOMAS

Immature teratomas contain elements that resemble tissues derived from the embryo. Pure immature teratomas account for 10–20% of all ovarian malignancies in women less than 20 years of age. Malignant transformation of a mature teratoma occurs in 0.5–2.0% of tumours, commonly to squamous cell carcinoma but, rarely, to adenocarcinomas, primary melanomas or carcinoid tumours. Immature teratomas are classified according to a grading system (grades 1 to 3), based upon the degree of differentiation and the quantity of immature tissue. Tumours with malignant squamous elements have a poorer prognosis.

Premenopausal women with disease confined to a single ovary are treated by unilateral salpingo-oophorectomy with surgical staging. Contralateral ovarian involvement is rare. Women with stage IA, grade 1 tumours do not require adjuvant therapy. All other stages are treated with adjuvant BEP combination chemotherapy (see also Chapter 8). Radiation is reserved for women with localised persistent disease post-chemotherapy (see Chapter 7).

The most important prognostic feature of immature teratomas is the grade of the lesion.[7] The overall 5-year survival rate for pure immature teratomas is 70–80%.

ENDODERMAL SINUS TUMOUR

Endodermal sinus tumours are derived from the primitive yolk sac. The median age at presentation is 18 years and approximately one-third of cases are premenarchal. Abdominal and/or pelvic pain occurs in 75% and 10% have an asymptomatic pelvic mass. Most endodermal sinus tumours secrete AFP, rarely, they secrete α1-antitrypsin.

The surgical treatment of endodermal sinus tumour is unilateral salpingo-oophorectomy, with frozen section for diagnosis. The addition of hysterectomy and contralateral salpingo-oophorectomy does not alter outcome.[5] Surgical staging is not indicated as all patients require either adjuvant or therapeutic combination chemotherapy with BEP or POMB-ACE. Survival has improved significantly with the introduction of routine combination chemotherapy, with 2-year survival now greater than 70%.

EMBRYONAL CARCINOMA

Embryonal carcinoma of the ovary is extremely rare and is distinguished from choriocarcinoma of the ovary by the absence of syncytiotrophoblastic and cytotrophoblastic cells. The median age at presentation is 14 years and women may present with signs of precocious pseudopuberty as the tumours may secrete estrogens. These tumours frequently secrete AFP and hCG. Management is as for endodermal sinus tumours: unilateral salpingo-oophorectomy and adjuvant BEP chemotherapy.

POLYEMBRYOMA

Polyembryoma of the ovaries is extremely rare, occurring in very young premenarchal girls. The tumour is composed of 'embryoid bodies', consisting of endoderm, mesoderm and ectoderm and secretes AFP and hCG. Chemotherapy with VAC (vincristine, actinomycin D and cyclophosphamide) has been reported to be effective.

CHORIOCARCINOMA OF THE OVARY

Pure non-gestational choriocarcinoma of the ovary is also extremely rare. Most women are aged less than 20 years and have metastases at presentation. Treatment is with chemotherapy but the prognosis is poor.

MIXED GERM-CELL TUMOURS

Mixed germ-cell tumours of the ovary contain two or more elements of the previously described germ-cell tumours. The most frequent combin-ation is dysgerminoma and endodermal sinus tumour. The tumours may secrete AFP or hCG, depending on the components. Treatment is with combination BEP chemotherapy. The most important prognostic features are the size of the primary tumour and the relative amount of the most malignant component. Stage IA lesions of less than 10 cm have a 100% survival rate.

OVARIAN SEX-CORD STROMAL CELL TUMOURS

Sex-cord stromal tumours account for 5–8% of all ovarian malignancies.[5] These tumours are derived from the sex cords and the ovarian stroma or mesenchyme, and include the 'female' cells (granulosa and theca cells) and 'male' cells (Sertoli and Leydig cells).

GRANULOSA–STROMAL CELL TUMOURS

Granulosa–stromal cell tumours include granulosa-cell tumours, thecomas and fibromas. The granulosa–stromal cell tumour is a low-grade malignancy. Thecomas and fibromas are rarely malignant and are they referred to as fibrosarcomas.

GRANULOSA-CELL TUMOURS

Granulosa-cell tumours secrete estrogen and occur in women of all ages. Five percent are found in prepubertal girls and are associated with sexual pseudoprecocity. In women of reproductive age, they present with menstrual irregularity, secondary amenorrhoea or endometrial cystic hyperplasia. Postmenopausal bleeding is a common feature, owing to estrogenic stimulation of the endometrium. Endometrial cancer occurs in at least 5% of cases of granulosa-cell tumour and 25–50% are associated with endometrial hyperplasia. Rarely, they may produce androgens and cause virilisation. They are bilateral in 2% of cases.

Granulosa-cell tumours may present like any ovarian tumour but tend to be haemorrhagic, occasionally rupturing and causing a haemoperitoneum. They usually present as stage I disease but may recur 5–30 years after initial diagnosis, with lung, liver or brain metastases. Inhibin is secreted by granulosa-cell tumours and is a useful marker for the disease.

Management

The treatment of granulosa-cell tumours depends upon the age of the woman and the extent of the disease. Stage IA tumours in women desirous of fertility are treated by unilateral salpingo-oophorectomy. In women not wanting fertility, a total abdominal hysterectomy and bilateral salpingo-oophorectomy is performed. If the uterus is left in place, a dilatation and curettage of the uterus should be performed to exclude a coexistent adenocarcinoma of the endometrium.

Adjuvant chemotherapy with BEP is used to treat recurrent or metastatic disease. Pelvic radiation may help to palliate isolated pelvic recurrences.[8] The 10-year survival rate for granulosa-cell tumours is greater than 90%; at 20 years, the survival rate falls to 75%.

SERTOLI–LEYDIG TUMOURS

Sertoli–Leydig tumours consist of Sertoli cells, Leydig cells and fibroblasts in varying proportions. They account for 0.5% of all ovarian cancers and are usually low-grade malignancies. Seventy-five percent occur in women less than 40 years of age and they often cause virilisation due to androgen secretion (oligomenorrhoea, breast atrophy, acne, hirsutism, clitoromegaly, deepening of the voice and temporal baldness).

Management is with unilateral salpingo-oophorectomy and evaluation of the contralateral ovary is adequate treatment in patients desirous of fertility. Older women are usually treated by total abdominal hysterectomy and bilateral salpingo-oophorectomy. Pelvic radiation and VAC chemotherapy have also been used in this disease. The 5-year survival rate is 70–90%.

Transitional-cell (Brenner) tumours of the ovary

Brenner tumours account for 1–2% of all ovarian tumours. They are bilateral in 10–15% of cases and commonly present in the fifth and sixth decades. They arise from wolffian metaplasia of the ovarian surface epithelium and consist of islands of transitional epithelium (Walthard nests) in dense fibrous stroma. Most tumours are less than 2 cm in diameter.

Brenner tumours are commonly benign but may be borderline and, rarely, malignant. Malignant Brenner tumours are defined by coexistence of a benign Brenner tumour component and a transitional-cell carcinoma. These tumours can secrete estrogen and often present with abnormal vaginal bleeding. The prognosis is good if the tumour is confined to the ovary.

Vaginal cancer

Primary carcinoma of the vagina accounts for 1–2% of gynaecological malignancies. Most vaginal carcinomas are secondary, usually from the cervix, endometrium, colon or rectum and, occasionally, from the ovary or vulva. Squamous-cell carcinoma is the most common type of vaginal cancer, with a mean age at presentation of 60 years. Approximately 9% of primary vaginal carcinomas are adenocarcinomas, which usually present in younger women. Vaginal sarcomas are extremely rare and are treated by surgical excision.

RISK FACTORS

Up to 30% of primary vaginal cancers occur in women with a history of preinvasive or invasive cervical cancer.[9] Vaginal intraepithelial neoplasia is known to be a precursor but its malignant potential is unknown.[10] The risk of clear-cell adenocarcinoma of the vagina in female offspring exposed to diethylstilbestrol in utero is 1/1000 between birth and age 34 years.[11] Approximately 70% of vaginal adenocarcinomas are stage I at diagnosis.

FIGO STAGING OF CARCINOMA OF THE VAGINA

Staging of vaginal carcinoma is clinical, involving examination under anaesthesia, with combined rectovaginal examination, full thickness biopsy, cystoscopy, sigmoidoscopy and radiological investigation (Appendix 1).

PRESENTATION AND DIAGNOSIS

Most women present with vaginal bleeding or discharge (Figure 13.3). Other symptoms include dysuria, urinary frequency, pelvic pain or pelvic mass and tenesmus. Careful inspection of the vaginal walls while withdrawing the bivalve speculum is required to identify the tumour, which is commonly present in the upper one-third of the vagina and easily missed on examination.

INVESTIGATIONS

- Full blood count
- Urea and electrolytes
- Liver function tests
- Chest X-ray
- Pelvic/abdominal ultrasound scan
- Intravenous urogram
- CT/MRI of abdomen and pelvis.

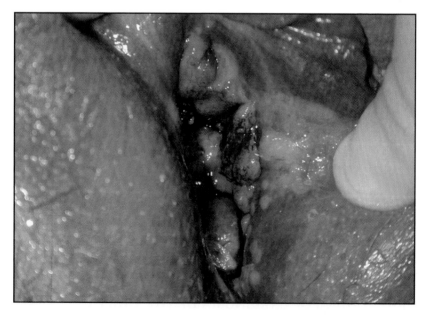

Figure 13.3 Primary vaginal cancer

MANAGEMENT

There is no consensus as to the correct management of primary vaginal cancer. Treatment is individualised and, for most women, maintenance of a functional vagina is important.

Radiotherapy

Most women are treated with radiotherapy, consisting of a combination of teletherapy (external beam radiotherapy) and brachytherapy (intracavity or interstitial therapy). The mid-tumour dose should be at least 75 Gy and complications occur in 10–20% of cases. Vaginal necrosis may occur and vaginal stenosis occurs in between 13–48%. If the lower one-third of the vagina is involved, the inguinal nodes should be treated or dissected.

Surgery

Surgery has a limited role in the management of women with vaginal cancer. It is considered in:

- Stage I disease involving the upper posterior vagina: involves radical hysterectomy, partial vaginectomy and bilateral pelvic lymphadenectomy
- small, low, mobile stage I tumours: involves vulvectomy with inguinal lymphadenectomy
- young women who require radiotherapy: pretreatment laparotomy allows ovarian transposition, surgical staging and resection of enlarged lymph nodes
- stage IVA disease, particularly if rectovaginal or vesicovaginal fistula present: pelvic exenteration may be appropriate
- women with a central recurrence after radiotherapy often require pelvic exenteration.

The complications of vaginectomy for vaginal cancer include:

- haemorrhage
- trauma to bladder or rectum
- fixity of bladder base: scarring of bladder base can fix the urethra causing retention or urinary incontinence
- loss of all or part of the vagina
- shortening and scarring of the vagina: may require skin grafting
- fistulae formation
- chemotherapy.

Combined chemoradiation has been used as first-line treatment for advanced disease and palliative chemotherapy for recurrent disease. Experience is limited and has included the use of 5-fluorouracil, mitomycin-C and cisplatin.[12]

OUTCOME

The 5-year survival rates for vaginal carcinoma is 64–90% for stage-I disease, 29–66% for stage II disease and 17–49% for stage III disease. The wide ranges in the reported 5-year survival rates are probably related to the small numbers of cases in the reported series.

Uterine sarcomas

Uterine sarcomas are mesodermal tumours and account for 3–5% of all uterine cancers. They are a heterogeneous group of tumours comprised of leiomyosarcomas, endometrial stromal sarcomas and carcinosarcomas. Not only are uterine sarcomas a heterogeneous group with regard to pathological features but they also have heterogeneous clinical characteristics. FIGO has only recently introduced a staging system for these tumours to separate them from the corpus uteri staging (Appendix 1).

RISK FACTORS

Uterine sarcomas are more common in black women and women who have undergone previous pelvic irradiation.

STAGING OF UTERINE SARCOMAS

See Appendix 1.

PRESENTATION AND DIAGNOSIS

Leiomyosarcomas usually arise *de novo* from uterine smooth muscle but 5–10% develop in a pre-existing fibroid, which may present with rapid enlargement. Women may also present with pain, abnormal uterine bleeding or a pelvic abdominal mass. Leiomyosarcomas can be diagnosed on endometrial curettage but more than 80% are diagnosed incidentally at hysterectomy.

Endometrial stromal sarcomas are derived from the stromal cells of the endometrium and account for 15–20% of uterine sarcomas. They are premenopausal in more than 50% of women and they usually present with abnormal vaginal bleeding. Low-grade stromal sarcomas have fewer than five mitoses per ten high-power fields and although they grow slowly, late recurrence can occur. High-grade stromal sarcomas, with more than ten mitoses per ten high-power fields, are aggressive tumours with an overall survival of less than 50%. Most are diagnosed at endometrial curettage.

Mixed mesodermal tumours (Figure 13.4) usually occur in post-menopausal women who present with vaginal bleeding and often the tumour is seen protruding through the cervical os like a polyp.

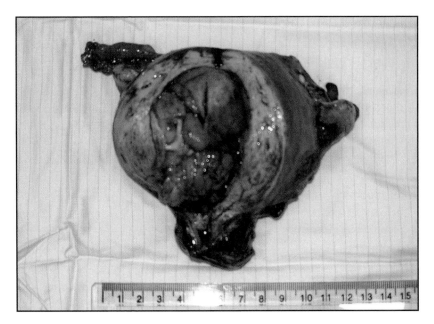

Figure 13.4 Mixed müllerian tumour

MANAGEMENT

Uterine sarcomas are treated by surgical excision. This typically involves total abdominal hysterectomy and bilateral salpingo-oophorectomy, but young women with a leiomyosarcoma may have ovarian preservation. Adjuvant radiotherapy is considered to improve tumour control in the pelvis and may improve survival in surgical stage I or II disease.[13] Complete response rates of up to 8% have been achieved with adjuvant chemotherapy with doxorubicin, cisplatin and ifosfamide.

OUTCOME

The 5-year survival rate for malignant uterine sarcomas is approximately 50%. There is no difference in 5-year survival rates for the three main histological types, when corrected for stage of disease at presentation.

Paediatric oncology

Gynaecological malignancy is uncommon in childhood and adolescence. If malignancy is suspected, girls should be referred to a gynaecological oncologist, owing to the rarity of the tumour. Neonatal cancers are usually embryonic tumours, with sarcomas presenting in adolescence.

OVARIAN TUMOURS

Ovarian tumours are the most common gynaecological tumours in girls but they account for no more than 1% of all tumours in girls under 16 years of age. About 30% of childhood ovarian tumours are benign teratomas. The most common malignant ovarian tumours in childhood are germ-cell carcinomas: dysgerminoma, endodermal sinus tumour, malignant teratoma and, more rarely, embryonal carcinoma, primary ovarian choriocarcinoma and mixed germ-cell tumour. Ovarian tumours in childhood present with:

- abdominal pain
- an abdominal mass
- urinary frequency
- rectal discomfort
- anorexia.

Treatment involves surgical excision by unilateral oophorectomy with pelvic and para-aortic lymphadenectomy when appropriate. Many tumours also require adjuvant postoperative chemotherapy.

UTERINE TUMOURS

Uterine tumours are extremely rare in childhood and adolescence.

CERVICAL TUMOURS

The most common tumour of the cervix and vagina in girls under 16 years of age is sarcoma botryoides, with 90% of girls presenting before the age of 5 years.[14] The tumour usually arises from the vagina in young girls and the cervix and upper vagina in older girls or adolescents. The mass is often grape-like in appearance. The majority of girls (80%) with sarcoma botryoides present with abnormal vaginal bleeding, a bloody vaginal discharge and a vaginal or abdominal mass.

Diagnosis is made by examination under anaesthesia and biopsy, which should include proctoscopy and cystoscopy. Multimodality treatment combining chemotherapy and radiotherapy with less radical surgery has enabled preservation of reproductive function in early stage disease. Chemotherapy alone with VAC can achieve a 'cure' in 82% of cases.[15]

VAGINAL TUMOURS

Clear-cell adenocarcinoma of the vagina is rare and is associated with vaginal adenosis and exposure to diethylstilbestrol in utero. The tumour is usually situated in the upper anterior third of the vagina and may be asymptomatic. However, it often presents with vaginal discharge and/or postcoital bleeding. Early disease can be treated by wide local excision, lymphadenectomy and adjuvant radiotherapy, whereas more advanced disease requires radical surgery and adjuvant radiotherapy.

VULVAL TUMOURS

Vulval tumours are extremely rare in childhood and adolescence. These include squamous cell carcinoma, malignant melanomas and sarcoma botryoides.

References

1. Curry SL, Schlaerth JB, Kohorn EI, Boyce JB, Gore H, Twiggs LB, et al. Hormonal contraception and trophoblastic sequelae after hydatidiform mole (a Gynecologic Oncology Group study). Am J Obstet Gynecol 1989;160:805–11.

2. Bagshawe KD. Risk and prognostic factors in trophoblastic neoplasia. Cancer 1976;38:1373–85.

3. Berkowitz RS, Im SS, Bernstein MR, Goldstein DP. Gestational trophoblastic disease: subsequent pregnancy outcome, including repeat molar pregnancy. J Reprod Med 1998;43:81–6.

4. Podratz KC, Podczaski ES, Gaffey TA, O'Brien PC, Schray MF, Malkasian GD. Primary carcinoma of the fallopian tube. Am J Obstet Gynecol 1986;154:1319–26.

5. Gershenson DM. Management of early ovarian cancer: germ cell and sex-cord stromal tumours. Gynecol Oncol 1994;55:S62–S72.

6. Gershenson DM. Update on malignant ovarian germ cell tumours. Cancer 1993;71:1581–90.

7. O'Connor DM, Norris HJ. The influence of grade on the outcome of stage I ovarian immature (malignant) teratomas and the reproducibility of grading. Int J Gynecol Pathol 1994;13:283–9.

8. Segal R, DePetrillo AD, Thomas G. Clinical review of adult granulose cell tumours of the ovary. Gynecol Oncol 1995;56:338–44.

9. Rubin SC, Young J, Mikuta JJ. Squamous carcinoma of the vagina: treatment, complications, and long-term follow-up. Gynecol Oncol 1985;20:346–53.

10. Benedet JL, Saunders BH. Carcinoma in situ of the vagina. Am J Obstet Gynecol 1984;148:695–700.

11. Melnick S, Cole P, Anderson D, Herbst A. Rates and risks of diethylstilboestrol related to clear cell adenocarcinoma of the vagina and cervix. Cancer 1996;79:2229–36.

12. Kirkbride P, Fyles A, Rawlings GA, Manchul L, Levin W, Murphy KJ, et al. Carcinoma of the vagina – experience at the Princess Margaret Hospital (1974–1989). Gynecol Oncol 1995;56:435–43.

13. Knocke TH, Kucera H, Dotfler D, Pokrajac B, Potter R. Results of post-operative radiotherapy in the treatment of sarcoma of the corpus uteri. Cancer 1998;83:1972–9.

14. Copeland LJ, Gershenson DM, Saul PB, Sneige N, Stringer CA, Edwards CL. Sarcoma botryoides of the female genital tract. *Obstet Gynecol* 1985;66:262–6.

15. Raney RB, Crist WM, Maurer HM, Foulkes MA. Prognosis of children with soft tissue sarcoma who relapse after achieving a complete response. *Cancer* 1983;52:44–50.

14 Palliative care

Introduction

Approximately 40% of the 17 000 women diagnosed with gynaecological cancer in the UK each year will eventually die from their disease. The principles of palliative care form an important part of disease management and are encouraged as part of good practice for all health professionals caring for these women. Where problems are more complex, persistent or difficult to manage, referral to specialist palliative care is recommended.

The World Health Organization defines palliative care as improving the quality of life of patients and families who face life-threatening illness by providing pain and symptom relief and spiritual and psychological support, from diagnosis through to the end of life and into bereavement. Palliative care:

- provides relief from pain and other distressing symptoms
- affirms life but regards dying as a normal process
- intends neither to hasten nor postpone death
- integrates the psychological and spiritual aspects of patient care
- offers a support system to help people to live as actively as possible until death
- offers a support system to help family cope during the patient's illness and in bereavement
- uses a team approach
- aims to enhance quality of life and may also positively influence the course of the illness
- may be valuable early in the course of the illness in conjunction with other therapies that are intended to prolong life (these include chemotherapy or radiotherapy and those investigations needed to better understand and manage distressing clinical complications)
- puts an emphasis on open and honest communication
- respects autonomy and choice.

In the UK, the introduction of gynaecological cancer multidisciplinary teams has greatly improved decision making and coordination of care for this group of women. Within the multidisciplinary team, the gynaecological cancer nurse specialist plays a pivotal role in supporting women and their families through diagnosis and treatment, sharing information with primary care teams and liaising with specialist palliative care services. Most specialist palliative care teams in the UK consist of, or have access to, medical, nursing, pharmacy, social work, physiotherapy, occupational therapy, complementary therapy, lymphoedema and chaplaincy staff. The service will usually consist of a hospital team, a hospice inpatient unit and a community team. Their role is primarily to work alongside other specialties to provide advice, support and education, although hospice inpatient wards allow more direct management of complex patients when required.[1]

Communication skills and breaking bad news

Good communication skills play an important part in all medical practice and are now more formally taught at undergraduate and postgraduate level. In particular, breaking bad news is not easy and can be daunting and demanding. However, it is a skill that can be learned and having a structured approach to these conversations can help. One example framework is shown in Box 14.1.[2]

Symptoms

Symptoms will depend to a large extent on the site of the disease, which local structures are involved and whether there are distant metastases. For example, involvement of the bladder or rectum may cause functional disturbance, whereas pressure on or invasion of the nerve plexuses in the pelvis may lead to pain. Management of the common symptoms associated with gynaecological malignancies are discussed below.[3]

PRINCIPLES OF PAIN CONTROL IN CANCER

History and examination

Full assessment of the cause of the pain is integral to successful pain relief.[4] Patients often have more than one pain and different pains have different aetiologies. The perception of pain can be affected by psychological and emotional factors and pain can remain difficult to control if these factors are not addressed.

Investigation

In the palliative care setting, investigations should be targeted at finding the cause of the pain, to guide appropriate treatment; for example, an isotope bone scan to look for bony metastases. Unnecessary and inappropriate investigations which do not change management should be avoided.

BOX 14.1 EXAMPLE FRAMEWORK FOR BREAKING BAD NEWS

- Find time and a private place.
- Try to have someone else with you, such as a nurse or a relative.
- Check the facts before the meeting.
- Find out what the patient knows; for example: "What have you been told already?"
- Find out what the patient wants to know; for example: "Are you the sort of person that likes to know everything about your illness?"
- Give a warning shot that bad news is coming; for example: "I'm afraid the test results were not very good"
- Impart the news slowly and as simply as possible, checking understanding and gauging response along the way. Be prepared to stop if the patient becomes distressed.
- Avoid saying "There is nothing more that can be done". Do not lie but offer realistic hope of, for example, controlling symptoms, treating pain.
- Listen to concerns; for example: "What are your main concerns at the moment?"
- Encourage expression of feelings.
- Summarise concerns and give an opportunity for questions.

Leave the patient with a plan and offer availability. Most patients need further explanation and support.

Management

Cancer pain management may consist of drug and non-drug measures. With proper assessment and a logical stepwise approach to analgesic prescribing, at least 80% of chronic cancer pain can be controlled. Where pain is not responding to treatment, specialist advice from the chronic pain team or specialist palliative care team should be sought. Consideration should also be given to treating pain by other measures including surgery, radiotherapy or chemotherapy, where possible and appropriate.[5] Referral to a physiotherapist or occupational therapist is helpful where pain is movement related. Complementary therapies such as aromatherapy and acupuncture can provide additional benefit to the patient. Cancer related pain can be described as:

- visceral/soft tissue: this is usually sensitive to opioids so use of the analgesic ladder is recommended (see below)
- bone pain: often responds to non-steroidal anti-inflammatory drugs (NSAIDs) and is partly responsive to opioids; radiotherapy to the

painful area may be helpful;[6] intravenous bisphosphonates given as a monthly infusion can also reduce bone pain.[7–9]

- nerve related: may respond poorly to opioids and the addition of adjuvant analgesics may also be needed (see below); non-drug measures such as transcutaneous electrical nerve stimulation (TENS) machine or nerve block may need to be considered in conjunction with drug therapy.

Also consider other causes of pain in cancer patients:

- treatment related; for example, constipation due to opioids
- comorbidities such as diabetes, arthritis.

The main principles of cancer pain control are:

- 'by the clock': cancer pain is continuous and therefore requires regular analgesia at appropriate dose intervals
- 'by mouth': the oral route is the route of choice unless the patient is unable to swallow or there are concerns about drug absorption
- 'by the analgesic ladder' (Figure 14.1).

Adjuvant analgesics are drugs primarily used for indications other than pain but which can provide pain relief in certain situations. They can be used at any step in the analgesic ladder. Common adjuvant analgesics used in cancer pain management include NSAIDs for bone pain, pleuritic pain and hepatomegaly; corticosteroids for raised intracranial pressure, hepatomegaly and nerve compression; antidepressants and anticonvulsants for neuropathic pain due to nerve damage or compression, and tenesmus; bisphosphonates for bone pain due to metastatic disease.

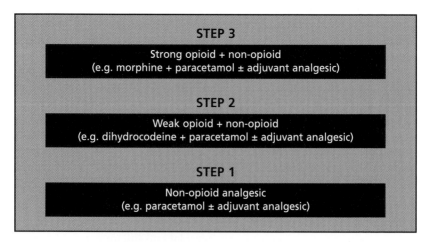

Figure 14.1 The analgesic ladder

When using strong opioids, it is important to establish initial pain control using immediate-release morphine at a starting dose of 5–10 mg every 4 hours (six doses daily) and titrate against pain with a 30–50% increase in total dose every 2–3 days if pain remains uncontrolled. Pain should be reassessed daily if possible. Once pain is controlled, maintenance therapy with 12-hourly modified-release morphine can be commenced. The dose is calculated by dividing the total 24-hour morphine dose by two. For example, 10 mg of immediate-release oral morphine every 4 hours adds up to 60 mg daily. This converts to 30 mg modified-release morphine twice daily. Although the regular immediate-release morphine is stopped at this point, a breakthrough dose of one-sixth of the 24-hour morphine dose (10 mg in this case) should still be prescribed. Other strong opioids may be considered if the patient develops unacceptable adverse effects on morphine. For example, fentanyl causes less opioid-induced constipation than morphine and is more suitable in renal failure. Advice should be sought from the specialist palliative care team if pain is unrelieved or the patient has unacceptable adverse effects.

Common adverse effects of opioids, both strong and weak, are constipation, sedation and nausea. Constipation must be anticipated and prevented in all patients on opioids. A regular laxative should always be prescribed when commencing opioids (see constipation section). Sedation may occur with the first few doses but usually lessens over time. Warning the patient and family that it may occur is usually sufficient. Nausea is a problem in approximately two-thirds of patients commenced on opioids. If it occurs, haloperidol, domperidone, cyclizine or metoclopramide may relieve nausea.

PRINCIPLES FOR CONTROL OF NAUSEA AND VOMITING

History and examination
Successful treatment of nausea and vomiting depends on identifying any potentially reversible causes, such as malignant ascites, and targeting antiemetic treatment towards the potential causes of the symptom. The patient should be fully assessed with this in mind. Potential causes for nausea and vomiting include drugs, renal failure, abnormal liver enzymes, hypercalcaemia, ascites, bowel obstruction, constipation, brain metastases, sepsis and humoral tumour effects.

Investigation
Consider requesting full blood count, serum urea and electrolytes, liver function tests, corrected calcium, plain abdominal film, abdominal ultrasound scan and computed tomography (CT) of the head, depending on the suspected cause.

Table 14.1 Drugs for nausea and vomiting

Cause	Drug of choice
Drug induced or biochemical	Metoclopramide, haloperidol, cyclizine or levomepromazine
Squashed stomach from ascites or hepatomegaly and delayed gastric emptying	Metoclopramide or domperidone
Stimulation of gastrointestinal receptors (e.g. local tumour, oropharyngeal candida, bowel obstruction)	Cyclizine or levomepromazine
Central causes (e.g. raised intracranial pressure, vestibular or motion related)	Cyclizine
Brain metastases	Dexamethasone
Chemotherapy induced	Ondansetron or granisetron (note: the place of $5HT_3$ receptor antagonists outside of chemotherapy induced nausea and vomiting and possibly post surgery is not proven. They can cause severe constipation and should not be used first or second line for other types of nausea and vomiting)

Management

General measures, such as providing smaller portions of food more frequently and avoidance of food with a strong odour, can be helpful. Stop or change drugs which may be causing nausea and avoid any drugs with anti-cholinergic effects if gastric stasis is present (hyoscine, anti-depressants, cyclizine). Where possible, abnormal biochemistry, including hypercalcaemia, should be corrected.

When prescribing antiemetics (Table 14.1), it is important to ensure that the chosen drug is prescribed regularly and to a maximum dose before changing to a different one. If the first drug is ineffective, change to a drug from a different pharmacological group. If the first drug is partially effective, a drug from a different pharmacological group can be added, for example adding haloperidol to cyclizine. Cyclizine and other drugs with anticholinergic effects will antagonise the prokinetic action of metoclopramide and domperidone. This combination should be avoided if possible. If symptoms persist for more than 24–48 hours despite regular oral antiemetics, drugs should be given parenterally. Where symptoms still persist, advice from the specialist palliative care team may be helpful.

MANAGEMENT OF MALIGNANT INTESTINAL OBSTRUCTION

Around 25% of women with advanced ovarian cancer develop bowel obstruction and surgical or medical palliative treatment can be used.[10] The onset is usually insidious, with repeated admissions for presumed subacute obstruction.[11] Clinical features include abdominal pain and distension, vomiting, colic, constipation and loud bowel sounds. Surgery should always be considered but may not be indicated or desired. The main principles of management are to control nausea, colic and other abdominal pain. It may be possible to keep a patient tolerably symptom controlled (although some vomiting may still occur) with medication given via a syringe driver and without a nasogastric tube or intravenous fluids (Table 14.2). In subacute obstruction, particularly if it is functional, a combination of metoclopramide and dexamethasone may be effective in restoring function. A Cochrane review of steroid use in bowel obstruction showed that they help to reduce inflammation but with no overall survival benefit.[12] Generally, when complete intestinal obstruction occurs, prokinetic agents such as metoclopramide and stimulant laxatives are to be avoided. Patients may be able to tolerate small amounts of food and fluid if nausea is well controlled. If large-volume vomits persist after a trial of hyoscine butylbromide (Buscopan®, Boehringer Ingelheim), a proton pump inhibitor can reduce the volume of gastric secretions. The somatostatin analogue octreotide may also be helpful to reduce gastric secretions.[13,14] Dry mouth can be managed with good oral care and ice to suck. If thirst is severe, intravenous or subcutaneous fluids can be used. Nasogastric tube or drainage gastrostomy may be considered, in discussion with the patient, to reduce symptoms if other measures fail.[15]

Table 14.2 Drugs used in a syringe driver for management of intestinal obstruction

Symptom	Drug
Abdominal pain	Morphine (starting dose 5–10 mg/24 hours or 50% of total oral 24-hour dose) Diamorphine (starting dose 5–10 mg/24 hours or 1/3 of total oral 24-hour dose)
Nausea	Haloperidol (2.5–5.0 mg) ± cyclizine (150 mg/24 hours)[a] or levomepromazine alone (starting dose 6.25 mg/24 hours)
Colic and to reduce secretions	Hyoscine butylbromide 60–120 mg/24 hours[a] Second line: octreotide (range 300–600 micrograms/24 hours)

[a] Do not mix cyclizine and hyoscine butylbromide in a syringe driver, as they may precipitate

CONSTIPATION

Constipation can be defined as difficult or painful defaecation and is associated with infrequent bowel evacuations and small hard faeces. It is common in patients with advanced cancer.

History and examination

Contributory factors include immobility, reduced oral intake, constipating drugs and raised serum calcium. Constipation should be anticipated in all patients taking opioids, $5HT_3$-receptor antagonists, or anticholinergic drugs (such as cyclizine or tricyclic antidepressants). Chronic constipation can cause anorexia, vomiting, colic, tenesmus, overflow diarrhoea, urinary retention and mental confusion.

Abdominal examination may reveal hard faecal material in the descending and sigmoid colon. Examination should include a rectal examination to guide management. In addition to determining the presence or absence of faeces and its consistency, it will also reveal any palpable tumour that may be exacerbating the problem.

Investigation

Measurement of serum urea and electrolytes will confirm any dehydration, hypokalaemia due to diuretics or hypercalcaemia. Plain abdominal film should not be used to diagnose constipation but may be helpful to confirm dilated loops of bowel if bowel obstruction is suspected.

Management

Constipation is a common cause of distress and is better anticipated and avoided where possible. Laxatives are the main treatment for constipation in palliative care patients but high fluid intake, fruit and fruit juice (particularly prune juice) can all help. Laxatives should always be started as soon as strong or weak opioids are prescribed. Laxative dose should be increased as the dose of opioid is increased.[16] A good first choice is the combination of a stimulant laxative with a softener such as senna and docusate sodium, unless bowel obstruction is suspected, when stimulant laxatives should be avoided. A laxative such as co-danthramer contains both stimulant and softening agents and can help to keep medications to a minimum. Patient should be warned that the dantron in this preparation stains urine red. It should be avoided in the incontinent patient as it can cause perianal skin irritation. Its use is restricted to constipation in terminally ill patients only, as rodent studies indicate potential carcinogenic risk. Movicol® (Norgine) can be useful as it is an osmotic laxative which increases the amount of water in the large bowel by retaining the fluid that it is administered with.

Lactulose alone is not usually effective in opioid-induced constipation. It should be avoided in patients with inadequate fluid intake and can cause flatulence and abdominal cramps. It is rarely necessary to use strong stimulant laxatives such as sodium picosulphate. Bulking agents are best avoided in palliative care patients as many are unable to drink adequate volumes of fluid and this can lead to faecal impaction.

Twenty-five percent of patients on regular laxatives will still need rectal measures at times. The choice between stimulant, osmotic or softening suppositories and enemas will in broad terms be governed by the consistency of the stool and how low down it is in the bowel.

DIARRHOEA

Diarrhoea can be defined as the passage of more than three unformed stools within a 24-hour period. It is a less common symptom than constipation in palliative care patients but can occur as a result of the constipation.

History and examination

As with constipation, patients can use this term in different ways and clarification of what they mean by it is always required. In women with gynaecological cancer, the most likely causes include over use of laxative therapy, drugs (for example, antibiotics, NSAIDs), faecal impaction with overflow, radiotherapy to the pelvis, colonic or rectal tumours and *Clostridium difficile*.

Investigation

Investigation should be aimed at finding a cause for the diarrhoea where possible but the patient's general condition will need to be considered. Specialised tests should be reserved for women with a longer prognosis.

Management

General measures include an increase in fluid intake and reassurance that most diarrhoea is self-limiting. Otherwise treatment will be targeted at the cause. If specific treatment is not available or the cause is unknown, opioids such as loperamide, codeine or morphine may be required.

RECURRENT MALIGNANT ASCITES

Ascites is the result of an imbalance between fluid influx and efflux in the peritoneal cavity. The healthy adult has about 50 ml of transudate in the peritoneal cavity. This has a protein level of about 25% of that found in plasma. Malignant ascites is an exudate with a protein content of about 85% of that found in plasma.

History and examination

Ascites can be asymptomatic when mild but distressing when severe.

Clinical features include abdominal distension and discomfort, early satiety, dyspepsia, acid reflux, hiccups, nausea and vomiting, leg oedema and breathlessness. In ovarian cancer, ascites is present in 30% of women at presentation and in 60% during the terminal phase of the illness.

Investigation

Blood tests, including full blood count, urea and electrolytes, liver function and international normalised ratio, are helpful prior to drainage. Abnormal clotting may need correcting prior to drainage and low platelets are a contraindication to paracentesis. Abdominal ultrasound scan will confirm the presence of ascites and allow marking of a drainage point. It will help to identify any solid tumour and also loculated ascitic fluid. A sample of ascitic fluid may be required for diagnostic cytology if ascites is the presenting feature of the woman's cancer.

Management

Chemotherapy may control ascites if appropriate and successful. However, if prognosis is poor and no further chemotherapy is possible, the principal of management in these patients should be one of minimal intervention. Unnecessary investigations should be avoided and for a patient who is bed-bound with a short prognosis, analgesia and good symptom control may be all that is needed. When a drain is inserted it should only be left in for a short period of time, usually less than 6 hours.

Paracentesis is appropriate for the symptomatic patient with a tense distended abdomen. The aim is to remove as much fluid as possible using a suitable catheter. Individual hospitals will have their own protocols but the following principles apply:

- Substantial ascites, as indicated by a tense abdomen and fluid thrill, can usually be safely tapped without imaging. As stated above, ultrasound can be helpful to mark an area for drainage if paracentesis has been difficult in the past or if solid tumour is easily palpable. Some centres now routinely insert drains under ultrasound guidance.
- 20 ml of fluid should be sent to bacteriology for microscopy and culture. In women where malignancy is suspected but not yet proven, the rest of the ascitic fluid should be sent to cytology for analysis. Ascitic fluid can also be analysed for protein content if the diagnosis is unclear.
- Clamping of drains to limit drainage rate is usually unnecessary, particularly for volumes less than 5 litres. There is some evidence that leaving the catheter on free drainage for 6 hours and then removing it is safe and effective.[17]
- The limited available evidence suggests that when draining 5–6 litres

of malignant ascites, significant hypotension is not usually a problem, the administration of intravenous fluids is rarely needed, and intravenous albumen has no role.

- Ascites will often reaccumulate and repeated paracentesis on an as-needed basis every 3–6 weeks is often necessary and appropriate. Diuretics may slow down the reaccumulation and may also be helpful if the patient has leg oedema. Spironolactone (starting dose 100–200 mg) antagonises aldosterone and can be used alone or in combination with frusemide (40 mg daily). Some units are now using semi-permanent catheters in patients requiring repeated paracentesis.[18] Peritoneovenous shunts are prone to blockage and therefore rarely used in malignant ascites.

LYMPHOEDEMA

Lymphoedema can be defined as tissue swelling owing to failure of lymph drainage.[19] In the UK, cancer and cancer treatments account for most cases of lymphoedema.[20] Combinations of two or more of the following factors greatly increase the likelihood of developing lymphoedema:

- axillary or groin surgery
- postoperative infection
- radiotherapy
- lymph node metastases (for example, groin, intrapelvic or retroperitoneal).

After radical hysterectomy for cancer of the cervix, including excision of the pelvic lymph nodes and postoperative radiotherapy, around 40% of women will go on to develop lymphoedema of the lower limbs.[21]

History and examination
Symptoms include tightness, heaviness, pain, impaired function and mobility, and psychological distress. Clinical signs include persistent swelling of a limb, which in time becomes non-pitting as a result of interstitial fibrosis and which does not decrease with elevation overnight.

Investigation
Other causes of oedema in malignant disease may need to be excluded (for example cardiac failure, hypoproteinaemia, salt and water retention due to drugs and pressure from malignant ascites). The following tests may be helpful if the cause is not obvious: full blood count, serum albumin concentration, serum urea and electrolytes and radiological imaging such as ultrasound, CT or magnetic resonance imaging (MRI) to determine disease status and to identify lymphadenopathy.

Management

The mainstay of management is good skin care with moisturising creams to avoid cracking and splitting. Avoidance of skin damage and aggressive treatment of any infection that arises in a lymphoedematous limb are of paramount importance. Tightness, heaviness and pain may precede any measurable change in limb size and early referral to a specialist lymphoedema service for further management is advisable. This may include lymph drainage massage and specialist compression garments along with additional lifestyle advice and counselling.

Diuretics are rarely of value in lymphoedema unless there is a venous or cardiac component to the limb swelling or the swelling has developed or increased since the prescription of an NSAID or corticosteroid.

BREATHLESSNESS

History and examination

Breathlessness in cancer patients can be caused by the cancer itself, cancer treatments, general debility or unrelated comorbidities. Potential cancer-related causes include anaemia, pleural effusion, tense ascites, lung metastases, lymphangitis carcinomatosis, superior vena cava obstruction, pulmonary emboli, radiation-induced pulmonary fibrosis, chest infection and cancer cachexia.

Investigation

Appropriate investigations to identify the underlying cause will include blood tests and a chest x-ray. Blood gases and an electrocardiogram may be appropriate in the acutely unwell patient. Pulse oximetry will also determine whether the woman is hypoxic.

Management

Management strategies must be targeted where possible at reversing the underlying cause. Where this is not an option, general management principles can be applied. Reassurance and explanation of the potential cause of the breathlessness is essential. Drainage of a pleural effusion or tense ascites is appropriate unless the patient is very near the end of life. Oxygen may be helpful if the patient is hypoxic but in non-hypoxic patients there is anecdotal evidence that the use of a fan to promote movement of air across the face can be just as helpful. Involvement of occupational therapy and physiotherapy expertise can help the patient to cope better with their shortness of breath. This can be achieved by adaptation of the home environment and teaching of pacing and relaxation techniques to deal with the anxiety that breathlessness evokes. Pharmacological treatment includes the use of low doses of opioids and benzodiazepines. Oramorph can be started at a dose of 2.5–5.0 mg every 6 hours and titrated according to effect.

Diazepam at a starting dose of 2 mg twice or three times a day can help with anxiety but accumulation can occur and cause memory loss and lead to falls. Lorazepam is longer acting but can be used sublingually for rapid onset in panic attacks at a dose of 0.5–1.0 mg.

MALIGNANT FISTULAE

A fistula is an abnormal communication between two hollow organs or between a hollow organ and the skin. Fistulae in advanced cancer can develop as a result of the cancer itself, postoperative infection, after pelvic radiotherapy or a combination of these factors. Advanced cervical cancer is the most common cause of a fistula among gynaecological malignancies. The fistula may be vesicovaginal (Figure 14.2), rectovaginal (Figure 14.3), enterocutaneous or a combination of these.

History and examination

Fistulae are virtually always symptomatic and the patient will usually volunteer a history of passage of wind from the urethra or passage of

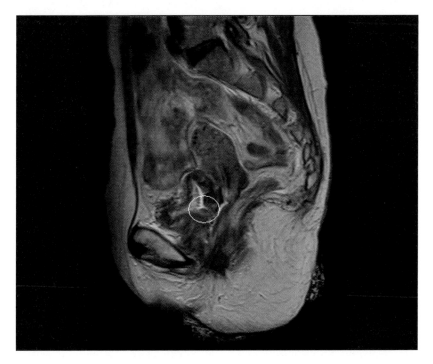

Figure 14.2 MRI showing a vesicovaginal fistula (ringed area; T2 weighted saggital image); courtesy of Dr L Gellet, Royal Devon and Exeter NHS Foundation Trust

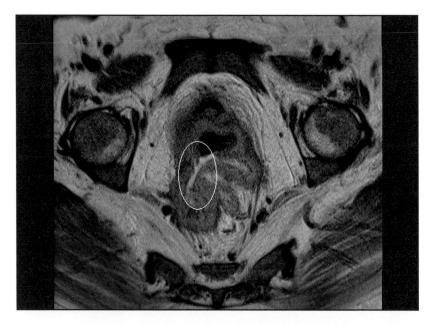

Figure 14.3 MRI showing a rectovaginal fistula (ringed area; thin section; T2 weighted saggital image); courtesy of Dr L Gellet, Royal Devon and Exeter NHS Foundation Trust

faeces through the vagina. In the case of a rectovaginal fistula, examination may reveal tumour or a palpable defect in the vaginal wall. The perineal skin may appear red or excoriated.

Investigation

Abdominal imaging such as a CT scan may be required to confirm tumour recurrence or in an attempt to identify the site of the fistula if further treatment is being considered. Barium studies may also be required. Radiological advice will help to determine the most appropriate investigation.

Management

A multidisciplinary approach to decision making and symptom management is recommended in these patients. This may include gynaecological oncologist, gynaecological cancer surgeon, palliative care specialist, continence nurse specialist, gynaecological nurse specialist and radiologist.

Fistulae can be distressing to women owing to discomfort, odour and loss of dignity. Surgical options should be considered for women with a reasonable life expectancy as this may significantly improve quality of life. Women with poor prognosis are best managed conservatively as stomas may not be trouble free and surgery inappropriate.

Conservative management will need to concentrate on urine collection using pads or tampons inserted in to the vagina, faecal collection using pads or stoma bags over an enterocutaneous fistula, skin protection with barrier creams, and odour control.

Surgical options will include urinary diversion, bowel diversion and fistula excision and repair. Formation of an ileal conduit, ureterostomies or occasionally nephrostomy may offer a significant chance of good palliation in those women requiring medium to long term palliation.[22] Where bowel diversion is concerned, the simplest possible operation is preferable although widespread intra-abdominal disease can make this difficult. Increasing expertise in colonic stenting may offer new and less invasive ways to manage patients.

TUMOUR FUNGATION

A fungating cancer is a primary or secondary tumour which has ulcerated through the skin. The tumour may proliferate or cavitate and is often associated with pain, pruritus, exudate, malodour, bleeding, infection and psychological distress to patient, family and carers.[23] Significant loss of self-esteem can occur, owing to effect on body image.

Investigation

If malodour or exudate is a particular problem, swabs will be required to rule out bacterial infection. Serum platelet levels and a clotting screen should be sent if heavy bleeding from the tumour occurs.

Management

Recurrent vulval disease, or occasionally cervical disease, can affect the tissues of the vulva, perineum and groin. Wide excision of such masses with or without skin grafting can provide useful palliation in selected cases. If the tumour is sensitive to radiotherapy or chemotherapy, significant reduction in tumour size can be achieved.[5]

Pain from fungating wounds can be multifactorial. Pain control should be approached as outlined above and will need to include drugs for neuropathic pain. In addition, there is some evidence for the benefit of topically applied morphine in the reduction of pain.[24,25] Nociceptive afferent nerve fibres contain peripheral opioid receptors which are silent except in the presence of local inflammation. Morphine is mixed with a water-based gel (such as Intrasite® gel, Smith & Nephew Healthcare Ltd), to produce a 0.1% (1 mg/ml) preparation. This can be applied directly on to the tumour twice to three times daily and kept in place by non-absorbable pads or dressings.

Pruritus is probably caused by inflammatory agents including prostaglandins and may respond to NSAIDs.

To control the exudate, specialist dressings can be chosen depending on the relative amounts of odour and infection. Malodour can be a particular problem and is caused by a combination of tumour necrosis and deep anaerobic infection. Treatment includes oral or topical metronidazole, charcoal dressings, occlusive dressings and sometimes debridement of devitalised tissue to remove the source of odour-forming bacteria using agents, such as topical Manuka honey. The patient may need to be nursed in a single room and the odour can be masked by using aromatic oil burners.

Surface bleeding can be controlled by application of adrenaline-soaked gauze (1/1000), silver nitrate sticks, alginate dressings and diathermy. Tranexamic acid in a dose of 1 g four times a day is a useful haemostatic drug that can be tried for persistent bleeding. Radiotherapy or embolisation may be needed to control more severe recurrent spontaneous bleeding.

Palliative care emergencies

Hypercalcaemia of malignancy is common in cervical carcinoma and is a poor prognostic indicator. Clinical features include anorexia, nausea, vomiting, constipation, drowsiness and confusion but it should be looked for in patients who are deteriorating with no clear reason. Although it often occurs in the presence of bone metastases, it can also be caused by secretion of parathyroid hormone-related protein by the tumour. Unless the patient is in the terminal phase of their illness, a persistently raised calcium level of greater than 2.8 mmol/l should be treated with intravenous fluids followed by intravenous bisphosphonates. Renal function will dictate safe volume of fluid and dose of bisphosphonate.

Massive haemorrhage is frightening for patient, family and staff. If the patient is thought to be at risk of a large bleed, a crisis pack of medication can be prescribed just in case. This would usually comprise midazolam 2.5–5.0 mg subcutaneously as required and morphine 5–10 mg subcutaneously as required (or one-sixth of the total daily subcutaneous dose calculated as above). Red and green towels should be available to soak up any blood. A reassuring presence is the most important factor and the patient may lose consciousness quickly. Always stay with the patient as the first priority, call for assistance and if a second nurse or doctor arrives, ask them to draw up and administer the crisis drugs.

Spinal cord compression should be considered in patients who develop problems with sensory changes or loss of motor function in the lower limbs. Urinary retention and faecal incontinence may also be presenting features. Spinal cord compression requires immediate commencement of high-dose steroids (usually dexamethasone 16 mg/day) followed by urgent MRI scan of the spine within 24 hours.[26] Advice from the oncology team regarding need for urgent radiotherapy or a neurosurgical opinion is advised.

The syringe driver

The syringe driver is a small, portable, battery-powered infusion pump which can be used to deliver medication by the subcutaneous route over a fixed period, usually 12 or 24 hours. It is normally reserved for use when other routes (oral, buccal, rectal or transdermal) are unsuitable or inappropriate. Local guidelines for use will usually exist. Although syringe drivers are often used at the end of life, they can be appropriate at other stages of illness.

Indications for use are: inability to swallow, persistent nausea and vomiting, interference with absorption via the oral route, and in the unconscious patient.

All of the drugs in Table 14.3 can be mixed with morphine or diamorphine in a syringe driver but it is good practice to avoid mixing more than three drugs in a syringe at one time, owing to the increased potential for drug interactions and precipitation. Cyclizine and hyoscine butylbromide should not be mixed in the same syringe as they may precipitate. It is important to remember to always prescribe as-needed doses of subcutaneous morphine or diamorphine for breakthrough pain.

Table 14.3	Drugs which can be mixed in a syringe driver		
Symptom	*Drug*	*24-hour dose in syringe driver*	*As-required subcutaneous dose*
Pain	Morphine	10 mg in opioid naïve patient or 50% of total oral 24-hour dose	2.5–5 mg hourly or 50–100% of 1/6 24-hour dose in syringe driver
	Diamorphine	10 mg in opioid naïve patient or 1/3 total oral 24-hour morphine dose	
Nausea	Cyclizine	100–150 mg	50 mg 8-hourly
	Metoclopramide	30 mg	2.5–5.0 mg
	Haloperidol	2.5–5.0 mg	0.5–1.0 mg 6–12 hourly
Sedative and antiemetic	Levomepromazine	6.25–12.5 mg	6.25 mg 6-hourly
Colic	Hyoscine butylbromide	80–120 mg	20 mg 4-hourly
Terminal secretions	Hyoscine hydrobromide (crosses the blood–brain barrier and is sedating)	1.2 mg	0.4 mg 4-hourly
Terminal agitation	Midazolam	10–20 mg	2.5–5.0 mg 4-hourly

The terminal phase

Optimal management of the terminal phase depends on recognition that the patient is dying. Signs that death might be approaching include the woman becoming bed-bound, only taking small amounts of food or fluid, becoming semi-conscious, and no longer being able to take her tablets. Communication of this fact within the medical and nursing team, to the woman's family and sometimes to the woman herself, is essential. It allows discontinuation of inappropriate drugs, unnecessary investigations and observations, and the prescription of appropriate drugs for symptom control.[27]

If the patient is unable to swallow, appropriate drugs for pain, nausea, chest secretions and agitation can be prescribed for subcutaneous administration as required. If symptoms are already present, the necessary drugs can be mixed in a syringe driver.

Some centres use an integrated pathway for care of the dying, such as the Liverpool Care Pathway, as the final multiprofessional documentation. These pathways aim to standardise care of the dying in all settings by applying evidence-based practice and appropriate guidelines.

KEY POINTS

- Palliative care forms an important part of disease management for women with incurable gynaecological cancer.
- Knowledge and application of the principles of palliative care should be part of the practice of all health care professionals.
- Where problems are more complex, persistent or difficult to manage, referral to specialist palliative care is recommended.
- Provision of palliative care to women with gynaecological cancer requires excellent communication and team working.
- Recognition that cure is no longer achievable should lead to a change in emphasis away from unnecessary investigations and treatment and towards comfort and good symptom management.
- Psychological, social and spiritual issues need to be addressed in order to achieve good symptom control.

References

1. National Institute for Clinical Excellence. *Guidance on Cancer Services. Improving Supportive and Palliative Care for Adults with Cancer: The Manual*. London: NICE; 2004.
2. Back N. Breaking bad news. In: *Palliative Medicine Handbook*. 3rd ed. Cardiff: BPM Books; 2001.

3. Herrinton LJ, Neslund-Dudas C, Rolnick SJ, Hornbrook MC, Bachman DJ, Darbinian JA, et al. Complications at the end of life in ovarian cancer. *J Pain Symptom Manage* 2007;34:237–43.

4. Hoskin PJ. Opioids in context: relieving the pain of cancer. The role of comprehensive cancer management. *Palliat Med* 2008;22:303–9.

5. Forbes K. Complications of radiotherapy for gynaecological malignancy. *Eur J Palliative Care* 1998;5:175–8.

6. McQuay HJ, Collins S, Carroll D, Moore RA. Radiotherapy for pain relief in patients with untreatable secondary cancer tumours. *Cochrane Database Syst Rev* 1999;(3):CD001793.

7. Urch C. The pathophysiology of cancer-induced bone pain: current understanding. *Palliat Med* 2004;18:267–74.

8. Gralow J, Tripathy D. Managing metastatic bone pain: the role of bisphosphonates. *J Pain Symptom Manage* 2007;33:462–72.

9. Wong RKS, Wiffen PJ. Bisphosphonates for the relief of pain secondary to bone metastases. *Cochrane Database Syst Rev* 2002;(2):CD002068.

10. Mercadante S, Casuccio A, Mangione S. Medical treatment for inoperable malignant bowel obstruction: a qualitative systematic review. *J Pain Symptom Manage* 2007;33:217–23.

11. Aletti G, Gallenberg MM, Cliby WA, Jatoi A, Hartmann LC. Current management strategies for ovarian cancer. *Mayo Clin Proc* 2007;82:751–70.

12. Feuer DDJ, Broadley KE. Corticosteroids for the resolution of malignant bowel obstruction in advanced gynaecological and gastrointestinal cancer. *Cochrane Database Syst Rev* 1999;(3):CD001219.

13. Mercadante S, Spoldi E, Caraceni A, Maddaloni S, Simonetti MT. Octreotide in relieving gastrointestinal symptoms due to bowel obstruction. *Palliat Med* 1993;7:295–9.

14. Massacesi C, Galeazzi G. Sustained release octreotide may have a role in the treatment of malignant bowel obstruction. *Palliat Med* 2006;20:715–16.

15. Brooksbank MA, Game PA, Ashby MA. Palliative venting gastrostomy in malignant intestinal obstruction. *Palliat Med* 2002;16:520–6.

16. Lakin PJ, Sykes NP, Centeno C, Ellershaw JE, Elsner F, Eugene B, et al. The management of constipation in palliative care. *Palliat Med* 2008;22:796–807.

17. Stephenson J, Gilbert J. The development of clinical guidelines on paracentesis for ascites related to malignancy. *Palliat Med* 2002;16:213–18.

18. Fleming ND, Alvarez-Secord A, Von Gruenigen V, Miller MJ, Abernethy AP. Indwelling catheters for the management of refractory malignant ascites: a systematic literature overview and retrospective chart review. *J Pain Symptom Manage* 2009;38:341–9.

19. Twycross R, Wilcox A. Lymphoedema. In: Twycross R, Wilcox A, editors. *Symptom Management in Advanced Cancer*. 3rd ed. Oxford: Radcliffe Medical Press; 2001. p.339–57.

20. Williams AF, Williams AF, Franks PJ, Moffatt CJ. Lymphoedema: estimating the size of the problem. *Palliat Med* 2005;19:300–13.

21. Werngren-Elgstrom M, Lidman D. Lymphoedema of the lower extremities after surgery and radiotherapy for cancer of the cervix. *Scand J Plast Reconstr Surg*

Hand Surg 1994;28:289–93.

22. Kochakarn W, Ratana-Olarn K, Viseshsindh V, Munangman V, Gojaseni P. Vesicovaginal fistula: experience of 230 cases. *J Med Assoc Thailand* 2000;83:1129–32.

23. Maida V, Ennis M, Kuziemsky C, Trozzolo L. Symptoms associated with malignant wounds: a prospective case series. *J Pain Symptom Manage* 2009;37:206–11.

24. Back IN, Finlay I. Analgesic effect of topical opioids on painful skin ulcers. *J Pain Symptom Manage* 1995;10:493.

25. Krajnik M, Zylicz Z. Topical morphine for cutaneous cancer pain. *Palliat Med* 1997;11:326.

26. National Institute for Health and Clinical Excellence. *Metastatic Spinal Cord Compression: Diagnosis and Management of Adults at Risk of and With Metastatic Spinal Cord Compression*. London: NICE; 2008.

27. Ellershaw J, Ward C. Care of the dying patient: the last hours or days of life. *BMJ* 2003;326:30–4.

Further reading

Ellershaw J, Wilkinson S. *Care of the Dying: a Pathway to Excellence*. Oxford: Oxford University Press; 2003.

Dickman A, Schneider J, Varga J. *The Syringe Driver: Continuous Subcutaneous Infusions in Palliative Care*. Oxford: Oxford University Press; 2005.

Hanks G, Cherny N, Christakis NA, Fallon M, Kaasa S, Portenoy RK, editors. *Oxford Textbook of Palliative Medicine*. 4th ed. Oxford: Oxford University Press; 2009.

Twycross RG, Wilcock A, Charlesworth S, Dickman A. *Palliative Care Formulary*. 2nd ed. Oxford: Radcliffe Publishing; 2002.

Twycross R, Wilcock A, Stark Toller C. *Symptom Management in Advanced Cancer*. 4th ed. Oxford: Radcliffe Medical Press; 2009.

Fallon M, Hanks G. *ABC of Palliative Care*. 2nd ed. Oxford: Blackwell Publishing; 2006.

Watson M, Barrett A, Spence R, Twelves C. *Oncology*. Oxford: Oxford University Press; 2006.

Internet resources

Information for professionals on drug prescribing in palliative care [www.palliativedrugs.com]

Website for national end of life programme: [www.endoflifecareforadults.nhs.uk]

Scottish Intercollegiate Guidelines Network (SIGN) guidelines on control of pain in adults with cancer: [www.sign.ac.uk]

15 Emergencies and treatment-related complications in gynaecological oncology

Introduction

Gynaecological cancers are more common in postmenopausal and elderly women. Most treatments in gynaecological oncology are instituted as elective procedures but acute presentations are not uncommon. Emergencies in gynaecological oncology are influenced by the site of cancer, stage of disease, presence of associated comorbidities and the treatment received. Emergencies can be medical or surgical.

Cancer-related emergencies

COMPLICATIONS RELATED TO ADNEXAL MASSES

Acute abdominal pain

The causes of acute abdominal pain associated with an adnexal mass are torsion, infarction, rupture and haemorrhage. Twisting of the ovarian pedicle results in torsion of the cyst causing a reduced blood supply, which leads to infarction and ischaemic pain. While smaller dermoid cysts are notorious for undergoing torsion, large tumours filling the entire pelvis rarely have space to undergo torsion. Infarction can also be caused by increasing size in a solid tumour resulting in diminished central blood supply. Rapidly growing tumours can develop internal haemorrhage by stretching and tearing of the feeding blood vessels or rupture of the cyst wall with bleeding into the peritoneal cavity.

Presentation

Patients usually present with sudden onset of abdominal pain radiating to the back and the thighs. Eventually, symptoms of peritonism (guarding, rigidity, rebound) and haemodynamic instability will develop with raised inflammatory markers and anaemia.

Management

If required, urgent normal crystalloid resuscitation and blood transfusion should be administered. Clinical examination should include general physical examination, abdominal palpation and a bimanual rectovaginal examination. Transvaginal ultrasound scan to assess the adnexa and any free fluid (blood or cyst content) in the pouch of Douglas should be performed. The use of tumour markers is not recommended as peritoneal irritation could result in false positive results. Laparoscopy or laparotomy to remove the adnexal mass is undertaken. In cases of torsion care has to be taken to identify and dissect the ureter as it can get entangled within the ovarian pedicle. Careful inspection of the peritoneal cavity for any suspicious deposits should not be forgotten.

COMPLICATIONS RELATED TO ADVANCED OVARIAN CANCER

Ascites

Approximately 75% of women with ovarian cancer present with advanced disease associated with ascites. Mechanisms of malignant ascites production are:

- increased capillary permeability by vasoactive factors (vascular endothelial growth factor, fibroblast growth factor, transforming growth factor) produced by ovarian cancer cells
- decreased fluid evacuation towards the pleural cavity caused by blockage of the lymphatic channels by cancer cell deposits on the diaphragmatic surfaces
- increases in ascites production by tumour cell deposits
- decreased intravascular oncotic pressure from loss of serum albumin into the ascitic fluid, which results in further fluid shift to the peritoneal cavity.

Symptoms

Patients present with shortness of breath, abdominal distension, discomfort, pain and indigestion. They may also have associated cachexia and signs of partial or complete bowel obstruction owing to miliary disease on the small and large bowel serosa.

Differential diagnosis

Medical causes of ascites (hepatic or cardiac origin, abdominal infections) must be excluded and large cysts filling the peritoneal cavity should be distinguished.

Management

The following steps are necessary in the management of ascites.

- detailed medical history
- physical examination, including:
  - abdominal examination to distinguish between ascites, omental cake, dilated bowel or a large cystic mass. The severity of ascites is assessed by detection of shifting dullness (moderate ascites) and fluid thrill (tense ascites)
  - rectovaginal examination to assess the pelvis
  - assessment of the chest to exclude an associated pleural effusion
- blood samples for full blood count, urea and electrolytes, liver function tests, serum albumin, serum CA125 and CEA tumour markers
- abdominal and pelvic ultrasonography to confirm ascites and mark the sites for safe ascitic drainage
- ascitic tap to relieve the symptoms and to establish the cause of ascites.

Rapid removal of large volumes of ascites does not have any adverse haemodynamic effect on the patient but those with poor cardiac status may require slower drainage with intermittent clamping and close observation. Intravenous access should be secured before drainage. The potential complications of drainage include drainage of a large cyst with intraperitoneal spillage of fluid, bowel injury, vascular injury and haemorrhage.

BOWEL OBSTRUCTION

Cancer-related bowel obstruction
A solitary tumour mass adjacent to the bowel or miliary tumour spread on the serosal and peritoneal surfaces may result in partial or complete bowel obstruction. Tumour masses on the large bowel with a competent ileocaecal valve can result in a dilated blind-loop. The increased intraluminal pressure will impair the blood flow in the bowel wall resulting in tissue hypoxia and necrosis and eventually leakage. Extensive serosal involvement by miliary tumour deposits leads to rigidity of the mesentery and the bowel wall. Bowel wall oedema associated with hypoalbuminaemia also causes multiple levels of intraluminal narrowing.

Surgery-related bowel obstruction
Bowel obstruction in the early postoperative phase is most commonly caused by strangulation due to adhesions or internal hernias or by excessive narrowing of the bowel lumen due to poor surgical anastomosis technique or oedema.

Signs and symptoms
Abdominal distension with colicky pain is usually the first symptom. Percussion of the abdomen is tympanic, the bowel sounds initially are hyperactive but in advanced stages they can be absent. Vomiting is common.

It is bilious with a dark green colour in the beginning but in advanced cases it can become feculent with light brown colour.

Diagnosis
Abdominal erect X-ray shows distended bowel loops containing air and fluid levels, with absence of air in the rectum. Contrast computed tomography (CT) may demonstrate the cause and site of bowel obstruction; for example, tumour mass, stricture. Blood examination for serum electrolytes is helpful to exclude hypokalaemia. A raised white cell count may support the presence of peritoneal irritation.

Differential diagnosis
Paralytic ileus also presents with abdominal distension, mild pain, vomiting and constipation. It is distinguished from intestinal obstruction by its early presentation (days 1–3) unlike intestinal obstruction (days 4–7). Clinical investigation confirms the absence of bowel sounds in ileus unlike the exaggerated bowel sounds in early stage mechanical obstruction. Abdominal X-ray shows generalised large and small bowel dilatation in ileus.

Management
Inserting a nasogastric tube relieves the stomach and reduces vomiting. Intravenous hydration with potassium supplementation is important, as patients are usually dehydrated and hypokalaemic, owing to intraluminal loss. Laparotomy and removal of the cause of obstruction should be considered in cases not responding to conservative management. If the large bowel is grossly distended (9 cm or greater) an emergency colostomy may be required.

If the cause of obstruction is surgically not salvageable (for example, peritoneal carcinomatosis) conservative management is advised: subcutaneous octreotide reduces the fluid production in the bowel lumen, while steroids help to improve the oedema. Introduction of total parenteral nutrition improves the patient's carbohydrate and nitrogen balance and the improved serum albumin level helps in reducing bowel oedema. If the patient shows a response to medical management and is fit, intravenous chemotherapy can reduce the size of the tumour mass and provide good palliation.

Palliative care and withdrawal of active treatment must be taken into account if the patient is not suitable for surgery and does not respond to the medical treatment.

COMPLICATIONS RELATED TO CERVICAL CANCER
Women with advanced cervical cancer may develop distressing symptoms and may present with acute admissions.

Pain from direct tissue infiltration or nodal enlargements impinging on the sciatic nerve can be managed with oral analgesics like acetaminophen, non-steroidal anti-inflammatory drugs (NSAIDs), oral or intramuscular opiates, transdermal fentanyl patches, nerve blocks or gabapentin for neuropathic pain.

Enlarged nodal masses or bilateral parametrial infiltration extending to the pelvic side walls results in bilateral ureteric obstruction and renal failure. Pre-renal and renal causes for failure should be excluded. The management of obstructive uropathy is dependent upon the general condition of the patient, her quality of life and the wishes of the woman and her relatives. The management of ureteric obstruction is controversial, as interventions to relieve ureteric obstruction may replace a peaceful death from uraemia with a painful, poor-quality life with marginally improved survival. Medical treatment options include either percutaneous nephrostomy, retrograde stenting or urinary diversions.

Women with advanced cervical cancer are at high risk of thrombosis from compression of pelvic vessels by the tumour mass, impaired mobility or effects of the treatment. Treatment with low-molecular-weight heparin is recommended if thrombosis is confirmed by Doppler ultrasound scanning.

An exophytic tumour can easily cause vaginal haemorrhage as a result of erosion of blood vessels. Invasion of the bladder or bowel can result in haematuria or rectal bleeding. Treatment is dependent upon the extent of bleeding: minor bleeding can be controlled by withholding any NSAID therapy, prescribing oral tranexamic acid, inserting vaginal packing or administering a single fraction of external beam radiotherapy. It is usually arterial and inevitably fatal in a palliative situation and therefore it is beneficial to forewarn the relatives or carers of a woman with advanced cervical cancer. If the patient is in a preterminal stage then the treatment is aimed at keeping her comfortable with sedation and anxiolytics such as midazolam.

Malodorous discharge can arise from a necrotic tumour, bowel or bladder fistulae. Oral or topical metronidazole reduces the odour.

Cervical cancer can erode into both the bladder and the bowel, resulting in fistulae with an associated offensive discharge, which can significantly reduce the patient's quality of life. If she is not suitable for exenterative salvage surgery then urinary diversion can be considered. Ileostomy or colostomy can be performed to relieve symptoms from bowel fistulae.

COMPLICATIONS RELATED TO ENDOMETRIAL CANCER

Vaginal bleeding from endometrial cancer can usually be managed conservatively. Intravenous administration of the fibrinolysis inhibitor, tranexamic acid, can be considered in cases of moderate haemorrhage. If conservative management fails or if the haemorrhage is profuse, emergency hysterectomy is advised if the uterus is resectable. In cases of advanced cancer invading the vagina, emergency external beam radiotherapy is required. If there is an associated pyometra, operative treatment for endometrial cancer should be preceded by intravenous antibiotic treatment to avoid septicaemia and other septic postoperative complications.

GENERAL COMPLICATIONS WITH CANCER PATIENTS

There are multiple causes for an increased risk of venous thromboembolism (VTE) in women with gynaecologic cancer: cancer-related thrombogenic factors; advanced age and limited mobility; compression of the pelvic vasculature by large tumours; lengthy surgical procedures; and chemo-therapy. The reported rate of VTE in gynaecological cancer patients is 15%.

Women usually present with painful lower-limb swelling, dyspnoea, chest pain and hypoxaemia. VTE can often be asymptomatic and may be diagnosed on cross-sectional imaging (for example, a thrombus in the iliac or lung vessels). The diagnosis of VTE is confirmed by venous Doppler ultrasound and CT pulmonary angiography. Immediate anticoagulation with low-molecular-weight heparin is required and if surgery is planned an inferior vena cava filter is inserted. Supportive care with oxygen therapy should also be instituted.

Complications related to surgery

INJURIES RELATED TO LAPAROSCOPIC ENTRY

Veress needle entry through the umbilicus has a potential risk of visceral and vascular injury. Visceral injuries include perforation of the bowel or bladder. Bladder injury can be avoided by emptying it before commencing the procedure. The only safe way to prevent bowel injury is to use Palmer's point when bowel adhesions are anticipated. Hassan open laparoscopy does not reduce the risk of accidental bowel injury but is the safe way to avoid injury to the large vessels. Careless direction of the Veress needle may lead to puncture of the common iliac vessels, aorta, inferior vena cava and external iliac vessels, in order of frequency. To avoid vascular injury, the direction of the needle in women who are obese should be perpendicular to the skin and angled at 45 degrees in women who are thin.

Accidental subperitoneal gas insufflation leads to surgical emphysema, which mostly resolves spontaneously within 48 hours. In severe cases, respiratory compromise may require omission of laparoscopy or conversion to laparotomy and postoperative ventilatory support.

VASCULAR INJURIES

Arterial injuries

The two basic forms of arterial injuries are blunt trauma and penetrating wounds. Blunt trauma to an artery can happen if continuous traction or compression is applied. Intramural haemorrhage and thrombus formation can result in luminal occlusion with subsequent distal ischaemia. Careful traction of the iliac vessels during lymphadenectomy can avoid such an injury.

Penetrating arterial injuries can be transections, lacerations and punctures. In cases of transection, mild-to-moderate haemorrhage and distal ischaemia are immediate consequences but the blood loss is usually not significant, owing to the constriction and retraction of arterial wall with clot formation. Arterial laceration usually results in more serious bleeding, as retraction of the cutting edge and contraction of the intact vessel wall will further open the wound. In smaller wounds, haematoma formation can provide some tamponade. Arterial punctures are spontaneously stopped by contraction of the vessel wall and thrombus formation. A false aneurysm can develop at the site of the weakened arterial wall.

Ligation of the internal iliac artery should be performed distal to the origin of the parietal branches, as bilateral proximal ligation of this vessel can result in gluteal claudication, owing to the reduced blood supply to the gluteal muscles. Ligation of the inferior mesenteric artery results in ischaemic changes in the rectosigmoid colon, so extreme care should be taken during para-aortic lymphadenectomy.

Immediate direct pressure has to be applied to avoid massive blood loss while transfusion of packed cells and crystalloids is arranged to allow for rapid fluid replacement. Adequate access for repair should be dissected around the vessel, following control of the proximal and distal ends of the injured vessel by vascular clamps. The distal arterial system should be irrigated with heparin to remove the distal thrombus and to prevent further thrombosis.

The type and extent of the lesion will determine the reconstructive technique. Punctures or small lacerations can be repaired using lateral suture of interrupted 5-0 or 6-0 polypropylene suture (or 4-0 for the aorta). Lacerations comprising more than 30% of the vascular circumference should not be closed this way to avoid stenosis of the vessel lumen: a widening patch should be used instead. Arterial transection can be repaired with a direct end-to-end anastomosis of the divided ends or an anastomosis using a graft placement.

Venous injuries

Veins are thinner and more fragile, owing to the lack of a robust muscularis layer, and their course is more variable forming plexuses and aberrant branches.

The course of the common iliac vein and close proximity to the artery makes it a common site of venous injury. Careful handling and dissection of the lumbar vein should be exercised during lymphadenectomy.

In 25% of patients, there is an anastomosis between the distal external iliac vein and the obturator vein (corona mortis or circle of death). Injury during pelvic lymphadenectomy can cause copious bleeding from both the external and internal iliac system.

A plexus of veins collecting venous blood from the pelvic muscles and organs – the pelvic side wall veins – can be injured during exenterative procedures or side wall resections.

In the distal inferior vena cava, 2cm from the common iliac junction, the precaval lymph node is attached to the inferior vena cava by a short and fragile vein: the Fellow's vein. Careless lifting of the lymph nodes may cause tearing in this vein, with significant bleeding. Owing to retraction of the vein, 4-0 or 5-0 polypropylene figure-of-eight stitch is required to control the bleeding following manual compression.

During mobilisation of the liver, careful attention needs to be paid to the hepatic veins draining into the inferior vena cava. Laceration of these veins may easily cause fatal haemorrhage. Before mobilisation, the inferior vena cava and the porta hepatis should be dissected and marked with rubber vascular strings to enable the surgeon to stop the hepatic blood flow.

Ureteric injuries

Ureteric injury is probably the most feared complication of gynaecologists, although a thorough understanding of retroperitoneal anatomy helps to prevent it. Ureteric injuries can occur during simple procedures by careless handling of tissues or attempts at haemostasis. The presence of a cervical fibroid, intraligamental tumour, pelvic side wall endometriosis or adhesions, malignant conditions such as cervical cancer and adnexal masses involving the side wall will make the ureters vulnerable. There are three high-risk anatomical sites in the course of the ureter where injuries usually occur:

- at the pelvic brim, where the ureter is in close proximity to the bifurcation of the common iliac vessels from below and the infundibulopelvic ligament from above
  To avoid ureteric trauma when the gonadal vessels are ligated, the retroperitoneum should be explored and the ureter visualised and palpated prior to ligation. Lifting the ovary away from the pelvic side wall also facilitates the safe ligation of the infundibulopelvic ligament.
- at the level of its crossing with the uterine vessels, the ureter is easy to damage with careless clamping. The uterine artery crosses the ureter from above while a number of uterine veins pass below

- the intravesical portion of the ureter is prone to injury during bladder mobilisation and during haemostasis following release of the ureteric tunnel during radical hysterectomy. Careful stitching or the use of bipolar diathermy during haemostasis prevents such injuries.

There are several types of ureteric injury:

- **deliberate:** during radical pelvic resection when malignant or benign conditions (endometriosis, ovarian cancer, sarcoma) are invading the ureter, part of the ureter may require resection. The ureter is intentionally transected during anterior or total exenteration when the bladder is removed with the surgical specimen.
- **accidental:** crushing trauma, needle trauma, transection, ligation, avascular necrosis.
- **delayed:** fibrosis-related stenosis, neoplasia-related stenosis.

Crushing injury of the ureter caused by clamping (with no transection) and needle trauma requires careful intraoperative inspection. If no signs of ischaemia are identified, retrograde stenting is advised to minimise the effects of transient ureteral wall oedema. However, if the crushing is prolonged or wide and the ureteral function fails to return, resection of the ischaemic area with end-to-end anastomosis may be required with ureteral stenting.

Complete transection of the ureter results in significant urine leakage and is usually identified intraoperatively. The ureteric ends need debridement and a retrograde ureteric stent is introduced immediately. The ureter is carefully mobilised to avoid tension and an end-to-end uretero-ureterostomy is performed using an oblique suture line to prevent subsequent stricture.

To avoid tension on the ureteric anastomosis, the bladder can be mobilised and sutured to the psoas muscle (vesicopsoas hitch). If the residual ureter is not sufficient for primary anastomosis, the tubularised bladder wall can replace a longer segment of the ureter (Boari flap). If the ureteric injury is close to the bladder ureteroneocystostomy is performed.

Partial transection of the ureter may remain unrecognised during the procedure. Patients develop fever, chill, pelvic tenderness or pain, abdominal distension, prolonged ileus, urine peritonitis and urine leakage from the vaginal or abdominal incision. Intravenous urogram or contrast CT is helpful to demonstrate the extravasation of the contrast material and to identify the site and extent of the damage. Depending on the patient's physical status, the extent of the injury and the interval since the operation, the management of partial ureteric transection can vary from insertion of ureteric stent to re-laparotomy and surgical repair. If the patient is septic and unwell, drainage of the pelvic urinoma with percutaneous nephrostomy helps to resolve the acute clinical situation.

Ligation or acute angulation of the ureter leads to hydroureter and hydronephrosis and presents with lower back pain, tenderness and fever. In the rare case of bilateral ligature, anuria is the presenting symptom. If the intravenous urogram or contrast CT confirms a complete ligation, emergency insertion of percutaneous nephrostomies is essential to avoid renal damage. Partially ligated or kinked ureter should first be stented with extreme care so as not to perforate the ureter. Subsequent surgical repair should be considered in cases of ligation. Occasionally, the injury is identified during surgery; the ligature then needs to be removed and the ureter closely observed. If no damage is identified, placement of a retrograde ureteric stent is required.

Avascular necrosis resulting in ureterovaginal fistulation is a rare complication of radical hysterectomy, when the blood supply of the ureter is impaired during its release from the ureteric tunnel. Women usually present with vaginal leakage 2–3 weeks after surgery. The diagnosis of ureterovaginal fistula is confirmed by the odour of the fluid, the raised creatinine level and the intravenous urogram. In most cases, conservative management with retrograde ureteral stenting is sufficient to reduce the symptoms of leakage and enhance healing. Occasionally, surgical repair is necessary with ureteroneocystostomy.

Bladder injury

Bladder injury is a frequent complication, mostly after previous caesarean section when the bladder is morbidly adherent to the uterus. In cases of muscularis or mucomuscularis injury, the bladder wall is closed in two layers using 2-0 Vicryl® interrupted sutures. Extreme care should be taken to avoid close suturing to the ureteral orifices. If in doubt, retrograde filling of the bladder using saline with methylene blue dye should be used to exclude leakage. During the early postoperative phase, overloading of the bladder should be avoided, so placement of a Foley catheter for 5 days is recommended.

Veress needle injury during laparoscopy may happen if the bladder is not emptied prior to the procedure. No action other than observation is necessary during the operation.

Bowel injury

Bowel injuries most commonly occur during debulking operations for advanced ovarian cancer. Needle injury to the bowel needs careful observation only in most cases with no suturing. Lacerations usually are sustained during sharp dissection of the tumour tissue off the bowel serosa, predominantly at the rectosigmoid colon or the transverse colon. En-bloc resection of the cancer with the adjacent bowel (Hudson procedure) and primary anastomosis should be performed to prevent bowel injury. If the bowel is lacerated and the edges are clear with no significant faecal spillage, primary closure with 3-0 polydioxalone interrupted suture is recommended.

The risk of postoperative leakage of rectosigmoid anastomoses is quoted at around 5%. Diabetes mellitus, hypertension, hypoalbuminaemia, smoking and previous radiotherapy are all important risk factors for leakage and defunctioning loop ileostomy should be performed to protect the anastomosis. Subtle symptoms such as low-grade pyrexia and abdominal tenderness with rise in white blood cell count may indicate an imminent bowel leakage. Frank leakage manifests as peritonitis with guarding, rebound and fever. When anastomotic leakage is suspected, full blood count and blood cultures should be taken and broad spectrum intravenous antibiotics commenced. Contrast CT can facilitate the diagnosis of anastomotic leakage by showing intraperitoneal collection or abscess. The cornerstone of the management is surgical exploration with consideration of revision of the anastomosis and bowel diversion (defunctioning ileostomy or colostomy) proximal to the site of leakage. Conservative management with percutaneous drainage can be considered in selected cases.

Bowel lacerations that are not identified during operation have identical clinical findings and management to anastomotic leakage.

Nerve injury

Nerve injuries are usually caused by transection or crushing impact by clamp or crude handling. Transection of the genitofemoral nerve during pelvic lymphadenectomy is not uncommon, mostly in patients who are obese, and this does not require repair. The patchy loss of skin sensation on the anterior thigh will recover postoperatively. During obturator fossa lymphadenectomy the obturator nerve can be damaged. In case of transection, end-to-end repair of the nerve is required. The adductor muscle function and some inner-thigh sensation will be lost but with active physiotherapy it returns in most of the cases. The sympathetic plexus can be removed during para-aortic lymphadenectomy, causing vasodilation of the ipsilateral leg so the contralateral leg feels colder. During Wertheim's radical hysterectomy, when the hypogastric nerves are not preserved, cutting through these structures results in impaired bladder innervation with difficulty in voiding. Routine use of either a Foley catheter or a suprapubic bladder catheter prevents over-distension of the bladder and ureteric reflux. This will also reduce the risk of ureteric fistulae. Nerve-sparing radical hysterectomy diminishes these complications.

EARLY POSTOPERATIVE COMPLICATIONS

Haemorrhage

Catastrophic haemorrhage after gynaecological cancer surgery is uncommon, owing to the extensive use of electronic haemostatic devices;

however, persistent oozing from large dissected surfaces may lead to haematomas. The use of biological agents such as haemostatic matrix (Floseal®, Baxter) or fibrin sealant (Tisseel®, Baxter) is effective in controlling oozing from extensive dissected surfaces. Massive, uncontrolled intraoperative haemorrhage from presacral or pararectal venous bleeding can also be controlled with packing of the pelvis and leaving the abdomen open (laparostomy). The packs are removed 48 hours later and the abdomen is closed.

Infection
The most common postoperative infections are urinary tract, respiratory and wound infections. Risk factors are obesity, diabetes, chronic obstructive pulmonary disease, malnutrition and immunocompromised state related to chemotherapy.

Thromboembolic events
Women undergoing oncological operations are at a significantly increased risk of deep-vein thrombosis or pulmonary embolism. Thromboprophylaxis with low-molecular-weight heparin, thromboembolic stockings, intermittent compression boots, adequate hydration and early mobilisation are mandatory measures to prevent thromboembolism. The presentation and management of thromboembolic events have been discussed earlier.

Paralytic ileus
Dehydration, electrolyte imbalance, prolonged surgery requiring small or large bowel dissection or resection predispose for development of paralytic ileus. Patients usually present on the second or third postoperative day with nausea, vomiting, abdominal distension and absent or sluggish bowel sounds. One should distinguish ileus from intestinal obstruction, which usually occurs later on postoperative days 5–7 and presents with similar symptoms and associated colicky abdominal pain and exaggerated bowel sounds in early stage. Plain erect abdominal X-ray shows generalised dilatation of small and large bowel loops. Management of mild paralytic ileus consists of intravenous hydration, correction of electrolyte imbalance and restricted oral intake. In severe cases presenting with profuse vomiting, nasogastric aspiration is required. Prokinetic antiemetics, such as metoclopramide, also facilitate resolution of paralytic ileus.

Shift in fluid balance
Shift in fluid balance is a special complication of debulking surgery for advanced ovarian cancer. Constant loss of protein-rich ascitic fluid during a prolonged operation usually leads to low serum albumin, fluid shift to interstitial space resulting in intravascular dehydration, fall of blood

pressure, impaired microcirculation and low urine output. Active fluid resuscitation with intensive monitoring of central venous pressure through a central line or with the recently advocated transoesophageal Doppler cardiac output surveillance is desirable for adequate recovery. There is no evidence supporting the benefit of using albumin infusion.

LATE POSTOPERATIVE COMPLICATIONS

Lymphoedema

Lymphoedema is often a presenting symptom of pelvic malignancies (adnexal mass, locally advanced cervical cancer, uterine sarcoma) which compress the side wall structures (veins and lymphatic vessels) (Figure 15.1). Postoperative lymphoedema is a result of surgical interruption of the lymphatic flow from the lower extremities, when lymph nodes are removed as part of staging or treatment. Underlying circulatory deficiencies, obesity, postoperative radiotherapy are risk factors for developing lymphoedema. Its incidence varies from 25 to 15% following radical operations. Most of the cases can be managed by active lymphoedema treatment and only a minority of the cases require management for long term complications.

Incisional hernias

Incisional hernias are more common with vertical extended laparotomies. Predisposing factors for hernia formation are multiple previous laparotomies, increased body mass index, elderly, chronic cough, constipation,

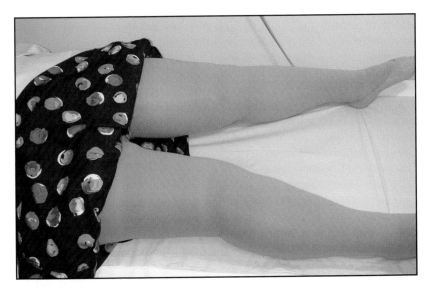

Figure 15.1 Lymphoedema

wound infection and poor nutrition, which all impair wound healing. The most common location for incisonal hernias is in the periumbilical region, as this is site with the least resistance and maximum strain. Presentation is dependent upon the size, site and contents of the hernial sac. Patients may present with an asymptomatic abdominal swelling or have symptoms of abdominal pain or even signs of intestinal obstruction. Hernias become a surgical emergency if they are non-reducible, if they have alteration of colour of overlying skin or they present with features of intestinal obstruction. The management of incisional hernias depends on the severity of the symptoms and can be conservative or surgical.

Complications related to chemotherapy

The most common complications which may require admission during chemotherapy are febrile neutropenia and vomiting.

FEBRILE NEUTROPENIA

High-grade pyrexia with a white blood cell count of less than 1000 micrograms/litre is a potentially life-threatening condition during chemotherapy. The nadir of neutropenia is usually on the tenth to fourteenth day after chemotherapy but, occasionally, a delayed nadir may develop. As their immune response is impaired, patients may develop severe infections with an inadequate inflammatory response: urinary tract infection with no pyuria, pneumonia with no typical symptoms. Patients on steroids may even lack the febrile response. Although the cause of infection remains unknown in 50% of cases, neutropenic patients with fever should be managed with a degree of urgency.

Careful physical examination, including the skin, oropharynx, perianal region, intravenous access or catheter sites and chest, as well as laboratory tests for full blood count, blood culture and urine culture, should be performed. Broad-spectrum intravenous antibiotic treatment should be commenced, which can subsequently be amended according to culture results. Consultation with the hospital microbiologist is mandatory. In cases of antibiotic-resistant sepsis, administration of colony-stimulating factors should be considered.

Nausea and vomiting are common complications of chemotherapy, especially of the highly emetogenic cisplatin. Administration of oral serotonin (5-HT$_3$) receptor antagonists (ondansetron, granisetron) is the cornerstone of the treatment, with additional low-dose dexamethasone and metoclopramide if necessary. The medications are better tolerated in rectal suppository format. In severe, cisplatin-induced vomiting, a natural killer 1 receptor-selective antagonist (aprepitant) is used with intravenous fluid infusion.

Complications related to radiotherapy

Complications of radiotherapy depend on radiation-related factors and patient-related characteristics. The total dose of radiation, the dose per fraction and the total volume irradiated are proportionately related to radiation-related complications. Factors related to the patient, such as previous pelvic inflammatory disease, history of smoking, diabetes, hypertension or previous pelvic surgery, will increase the risk of complications. Acute complications such as scalding of skin, diarrhoea and anaemia, are usually mild. Late complications can occur many months or years after treatment and are usually long-lasting.

- Bladder complications: radiation cystitis manifests as haematuria, frequency and dysuria.
- Bowel complications: radiation enteritis presents with severe diarrhoea, malabsorption, cachexia or bowel obstruction.
- Fibrosis of the pelvic structures results in reduced bladder capacity and pelvic pain. Fusion of the vaginal walls and shortening of the vaginal length results in dyspareunia and altered sexual function.
- Fistulae: rectovaginal or vesicovaginal fistula formation is a severe complication impacting on the patient's social life.

Conclusion

Prevention and timely intervention are crucial in the management of complications in gynaecological oncology. Owing to the potentially detrimental sequelae, input from senior clinicians is mandatory. Departmental registration and regular audit of complications are an essential part of governance and reduce the incidence of future complications.

Appendix 1:
FIGO staging of gynaecological cancers

FIGO has published revised staging systems for endometrial, cervical and vulval cancer and introduced a new staging system for uterine sarcomas in 2009.[1,2] The new staging system is in use in the UK from January 2010.

References

1. International Federation of Obstetrics and Gynecology Committee on Gynecologic Oncology. Revised FIGO staging for carcinoma of the vulva, cervix and endometrium. *Int J Gynecol Obstet* 2009;105:103–4.
2. International Federation of Obstetrics and Gynecology Committee on Gynecologic Oncology. FIGO staging for uterine sarcomas. *Int J Gynecol Obstet* 2009;104:179.

Carcinoma of the cervix uteri (2009)

Stage	Definition
I	**The carcinoma is strictly confined to the cervix (extension to the corpus would be disregarded)**
A	Invasive carcinoma which can be diagnosed only by microscopy, with deepest invasion ≤ 5 mm and largest extension ≥ 7 mm
A1	Measured stromal invasion of ≤ 3.0 mm in depth and extension of ≤ 7.0 mm
A2	Measured stromal invasion of > 3.0 mm and not > 5.0 mm with an extension of not > 7.0 mm
B	Clinically visible lesions limited to the cervix uteri or preclinical cancers greater than stage Ia[(i)]
B1	Clinically visible lesion ≤ 4.0 cm in greatest dimension
B2	Clinically visible lesion > 4.0 cm in greatest dimension
II	**Cervical carcinoma invades beyond the uterus but not to the pelvic wall or to the lower-third of the vagina**
A	Without parametrial invasion
A1	Clinically visible lesion ≤ 4.0 cm in greatest dimension
A2	Clinically visible lesion > 4 cm in greatest dimension
B	With obvious parametrial invasion
III	**The tumour extends to the pelvic wall and/or involves lower-third of the vagina and/or causes hydronephrosis or non-functioning kidney[(ii)]**
A	Tumour involves lower third of the vagina, with no extension to the pelvic wall
B	Extension to the pelvic wall and/or hydronephrosis or non-functioning kidney
IV	**The carcinoma has extended beyond the true pelvis or has involved (biopsy proven) the mucosa of the bladder or rectum. A bullous oedema, as such, does not permit a case to be allotted to stage IV**
A	Spread of the growth to adjacent organs
B	Spread to distant organs

[(i)] All macroscopically visible lesions (even with superficial invasion) are allotted to stage Ib carcinomas. Invasion is limited to a measured stromal invasion with a maximal depth of 5 mm and a horizontal extension of not > 7 mm. Depth of invasion should not be > 5 mm taken from the base of the epithelium of the original tissue: superficial or glandular. The depth of invasion should always be reported in mm, even in those cases with 'early (minimal) stromal invasion' (~1 mm). The involvement of vascular/lymphatic spaces should not change the stage allotment.

[(ii)] On rectal examination, there is no cancer-free space between the tumour and the pelvic wall. All cases with hydronephrosis or non-functioning kidney are included, unless they are known to be attributable to another cause.

Carcinoma of the endometrium (2009)

Stage	Definition
I[(iii)]	**Tumour confined to the corpus uteri**
A	No or less than 50% myometrial invasion
B	Invasion ≥ 50% of the myometrium
II[(iii)]	**Tumour invades cervical stroma but does not extend beyond the uterus[(iv)]**
III[(iii)]	**Local and/or regional spread of the tumour**
A	Tumour invades the serosa of the corpus uteri and/or adnexae[(v)]
B	Vaginal and/or parametrial involvement[(v)]
C	Metastases to pelvic and/or para-aortic lymph nodes[(v)]
C1	Positive pelvic nodes
C2	Positive para-aortic lymph nodes with or without positive pelvic lymph nodes
IV[(iii)]	**Tumour invades bladder and/or bowel mucosa and/or distant metastases**
A	Tumour invades bladder and/or bowel mucosa
B	Distant metastases, including intra-abdominal metastases and/or inguinal lymph nodes

[(iii)] Either grade 1, 2 or 3.
[(iv)] Endocervical glandular involvement only should be considered as Stage I and no longer as Stage II.
[(v)] Positive cytology has to be reported separately without changing the stage.

Carcinoma of the ovary

Stage	Definition
I	**Tumour confined to the ovaries**
A	Tumour confined to one ovary; capsule intact, no tumour on ovarian surface; no malignant cells in ascites or peritoneal washings
B	Tumour confined to both ovaries; capsule intact, no tumour on ovarian surface; no malignant cells in ascites or peritoneal washings
C	Tumour confined to one or both ovaries with any of the following: capsule ruptured, tumour on ovarian surface, malignant cells in ascites or peritoneal washings
II	**Tumour one or both ovaries with pelvic extension**
A	Extension and/or implants on uterus and/or tube(s); no malignant cells in ascites or peritoneal washings
B	Extension to other pelvic tissues; no malignant cells in ascites or peritoneal washings
C	Pelvic extension (2A or 2B) with malignant cells in ascites or peritoneal washings
III	**Tumour involves one or both ovaries with microscopically confirmed peritoneal metastasis outside the pelvis and/or regional lymph node metastasis**
A	Microscopic peritoneal metastasis beyond the pelvis
B	Macroscopic peritoneal metastasis beyond the pelvis $\leq$ 2 cm in greatest dimension
C	Peritoneal metastasis beyond pelvis > 2 cm in greatest dimension and/or regional lymph node metastasis
IV	**Growth involving one or both ovaries with distant metastasis[vi]**

[vi] If pleural effusion is present, there must be positive cytology; parynchymal liver metastases equals Stage IV disease.

Carcinoma of the vulva (2009)

Stage	Definition
I	**Tumour confined to the vulva**
A	Lesions ≤ 2 cm in size, confined to the vulva or perineum and with stromal invasion ≤ 1.0 mm,[1] no nodal metastasis
B	Lesions > 2 cm in size or with stromal invasion > 1.0 mm,[vii] confined to the vulva or perineum, with negative nodes
II	**Tumour of any size with extension to adjacent perineal structures (one-third lower urethra, one-third lower vagina, anus) with negative nodes**
III	**Tumour of any size with or without extension to adjacent perineal structures (one-third lower urethra, one-third lower vagina, anus) with positive inguinofemoral lymph nodes**
A1	With 1 lymph node metastasis ≥ 5 mm
A2	1–2 lymph node metastases < 5 mm
B1	With 2 or more lymph node metastases (≥ 5 mm)
B2	3 or more lymph node metastases (< 5 mm)
C	With positive nodes with extracapsular spread
IV	**Tumour invades other regional (two-thirds upper urethra, two-thirds upper vagina) or distant structures**
A	Tumour invades any of the following:
A1	Upper urethral and/or vaginal mucosa, bladder mucosa, rectal mucosa or fixed to pelvic bone
A2	Fixed or ulcerated inguinofemoral lymph nodes

[vii] The depth of invasion is defined as the measurement of the tumour from the epithelial–stromal junction of the adjacent most superficial dermal papilla to the deepest point of invasion.

Staging for uterine sarcomas

LEIOMYOSARCOMA

Stage	Definition
I	**Tumour confined to the uterus**
A	< 5 cm
B	> 5 cm
II	**Tumour extends to the pelvis**
A	Adnexal involvement
B	Tumour extends to extrauterine pelvic tissues
III	**Tumour invades abdominal tissues (not just protruding into the abdomen)**
A	One site
B	More than one site
C	Metastasis to pelvic and/or para-aortic lymph nodes
IV	**Tumour invades the following:**
A	Tumour invades bladder and/or rectum
B	Distant metastasis

ENDOMETRIAL STROMAL SARCOMA AND ADENOSARCOMA[(viii)]

Stage	Definition
I	**Tumour confined to the uterus**
A	Tumour confined to the endometrium/endocervix with no myometrial invasion
B	≤ 50% myometrial invasion
C	≥ 50% myometrial invasion
II	**Tumour extends to the pelvis**
A	Adnexal involvement
B	Tumour extends to extrauterine pelvic tissue
III	**Tumour invades abdominal tissues (not just protruding into the abdomen)**
A	One site
B	More than one site
C	Metastasis to pelvic and/or para-aortic lymph nodes
IV	**Tumour invades the following:**
A	Tumour invades bladder and/or rectum
B	Distant metastasis

[(viii)] Simultaneous tumours of the uterine corpus and ovary/pelvis in association with ovarian/pelvic endometriosis should be classified as independent primary tumours

CARCINOSARCOMA

Carcinosarcomas should be staged as carcinomas of the endometrium.

Gestational trophoblastic tumours

Stage	Definition
I	Tumour strictly confined to the uterine corpus
II	Tumour extending to the adnexa or the vagina but confined to the genital structures
III	Tumour extending to the lungs, with or without genital tract involvement
IV	All other metastatic sites

According to FIGO, hydatidiform mole should be registered but not staged as Stage 0 because, if human chorionic gonadotrophin (hCG) persists and the mother requires chemotherapy, restaging would be required. Such staging transgresses the present rules of the present FIGO staging system. Women with hydatidiform mole are placed on record but staging only applies to trophoblastic neoplasia.

Cases which do not fulfil the criteria for any given stage should be listed separately as unstaged. It should be realised that most cases of low-risk metastatic disease are contained within Stage III, while the high-risk group of metastatic tumours comes under stage IV.

In 2002, a modified World Health Organization (WHO) risk score was incorporated into the FIGO staging (page 253).

FIGO (WHO) risk factor scoring with FIGO staging[a]	0	1	2	4
Age (years)	< 40	≥ 40	–	–
Antecedent pregnancy	Hydatidiform mole	Abortion	Term	–
Interval months from index pregnancy	< 4	4–6	7–12	> 12
Pretreatment hCG milli-iu/MI	< 103	103–104	104–105	> 105
Largest tumour size including uterus (cm)	–	3–4	≥ 5	–
Site of metastases including uterus	lung	spleen, kidney	gastro-intestinal tract	brain, liver
Metastases identified (n)	–	1–4	5–8	> 8
Previous failed chemotherapy	–	–	1 drug	≥ 2 drugs

[a] a score of ≤ 6 is low risk; a score of ≥ 7 is high risk.

Staging for carcinoma of the fallopian tube (1994)

Stage	Definition
I	**Tumour confined to the fallopian tubes**
A	Tumour confined to one tube, no serosal penetration, no ascites
B	Tumour confined to both tubes, no serosal penetration, no ascites
C	Tumour confined to one or both tubes, with serosal involvement and/or positive ascites or peritoneal washings
II	**Tumour involves one or both fallopian tubes with pelvic extension**
A	Extension and/or metastasis to uterus and/or ovaries
B	Extension to other pelvic structures
C	Pelvic extension (IIA or IIb) with positive ascites or peritoneal washings
III	**Tumour involves one or both fallopian tubes with peritoneal implants outside the pelvis and/or positive regional lymph nodes**
A	Microscopic peritoneal metastasis outside the pelvis
B	Macroscopic peritoneal metastasis outside the pelvis not exceeding 2 cm in size
C	Peritoneal metastasis > 2cm in size and/or positive regional lymph nodes
IV	**Distant metastasis (excludes peritoneal metastasis)**

Staging for carcinoma of the vagina (1994)

Stage	Definition
I	**Tumour confined to the vagina**
II	**Tumour invades paravaginal tissues but does not extend to the pelvic wall**
III	**Tumour extending to pelvic wall**
IV	**Tumour invading mucosa of the bladder or rectum and/or extending beyond the true pelvis[ix]**
A	Spread to distant organs
B	Distant metastases

[ix] The presence of bullous oedema is not sufficient evidence to classify a tumour as Stage IVA.

Index

abdominal pain 215, 229–30
ablative therapy for CIN 46
acetowhiteness 43–5, 48
ACTION trial 107, 131
adenocarcinoma 20, 85, 99, 201, 206
adenocarcinoma in situ (AIS) 47
adenomyoma 22
adenosarcoma 251
adenosquamous carcinoma 20
adnexal masses 85–6, 229–30
   see also ovarian cancer
adverse effects *see* complications of
      treatment
age, incidence and 2, 4, 9, 115, 118, 190,
      193
analgesia 210–13, 215, 223, 225, 233
antibiotics 234, 242
anticonvulsants 212
antidepressants 212
antiemetics 214, 225, 240, 242
anus, spread of vulval cancer to 109,
      178, 182
aprepitant 242
arterial injuries, intraoperative 88, 234,
      235
ascites 58, 217–19, 230–1
ASTEC trial 62, 76, 85, 149

bad news 211
bevacizumab 132, 134
bilateral salpingo-oophorectomy *see*
      oophorectomy
biopsy 15–16, 67
   cervical 46, 157–8
   endometrial 146–7
   vulval 77, 171–3
bisphosphonates 212, 224
bladder, complications 75, 97, 238, 239

bleeding
   in advanced disease 224, 233, 233–4
   intra- and postoperative 75, 91, 235–6,
      239–40
   postcoital 156
   postmenopausal 4, 145, 146, 200
bleomycin 108, 110, 118, 198
bone pain 211–12
bowel injuries during surgery 231, 234,
      238–9
bowel obstruction 58, 70, 215, 231–2
brachytherapy 95, 96–7, 100
BRCA1/BRCA2 genotype 7, 137–8
breathlessness 220–1
Brenner tumours 201

CA125 85, 120, 121, 135, 136, 194
carboplatin 106, 131, 133, 162, 195
carcinoma in situ (CIS) 35
carcinosarcoma (mixed müllerian
      tumours) 22, 63, 146, 204, 251
cervical cancer 155–65
   chemotherapy 60, 107–8, 111, 162,
      164, 165
   complications of advanced disease 219,
      221–3, 224, 232–3
   diagnosis 46, 156–8
   epidemiology 1–3, 155
   follow-up 163–4
   imaging 58–62, 158, 159
   multidisciplinary teams in 155, 163
   paediatric 206
   pathology 19–20, 32, 35–6, 47
   preinvasive disease 16–19, 35–40, 43–6
   presentation 41–5, 155–6
   radiotherapy 61–2, 97, 98–9, 161–2,
      165
   recurrence 62, 73, 108, 164–5
   screening programme 40–6, 156

staging 19, 71–2, 158–9, 246
   surgery 72–4, 83–4, 160–1, 162–3, 164
   vaccination for HPV 38–9
cervical glandular intraepithelial neoplasia
     (CGIN) 17–18, 32, 47
cervical intraepithelial neoplasia (CIN)
     16–17, 35–6, 43–6
chemoradiation 103
   cervical cancer 108, 162, 164
   vulval cancer 100, 109, 111, 182
chemotherapy 103–11
   cervical cancer 60, 107–8, 111, 162,
     165
   complications 104–5, 106, 108, 242
   endometrial cancer 103–4, 109, 111,
     150
   fallopian tube cancer 195
   GTD 109–10, 192–3
   ovarian cancer
     epithelial 71, 106–7, 111, 130–4,
      135–6
     nonepithelial 110, 118, 198, 199,
      200
   vaginal cancer 203
   see also chemoradiation
choriocarcinoma 190, 199
CHORUS trial 107, 130
cisplatin
   cervical cancer 108, 162, 165
   complications 242
   endometrial cancer 109
   ovarian cancer 106, 110, 118, 198
   vulval cancer 109
clear-cell cancers 99, 150, 201, 206–7
co-danthramer 216
colostomy 182, 223, 232
colposcopy 42–6, 156
communication skills 210, 211, 226
complications of treatment
   chemotherapy 104–5, 106, 108, 242
   radiotherapy 62, 97–8, 150, 161, 243
   surgery 68–9, 70, 74, 75, 91, 130, 184,
     203, 231, 234–42
computed tomography (CT) 55–8, 60,
     61, 63, 65, 135–6
cone biopsy/excision 46, 83, 160
constipation 213, 216–17
contraceptive use 3, 4, 8
corticosteroids 212, 215, 224

cyclizine 214, 225
cyclophosphamide 106, 110
cytological screening 40–2, 156

death
   mortality rates 1, 2, 3, 6, 9
   terminal care 226
DESKTOP trial 134
diabetes mellitus 5
diagnosis 15–16, 29–30, 67
   cervical cancer 46, 156–8
   endometrial cancer 62, 145, 146–8
   fallopian tube cancer 193–4
   GTD 191
   ovarian cancer
     epithelial 30–1, 53–5, 85–6, 119–21,
      123
     nonepithelial 197, 200
   uterine sarcoma 204
   vaginal cancer 202
   vulval cancer 77, 170–3
diamorphine 215, 225
diarrhoea 217
diazepam 221
diet 3
diethylstilbestrol 49–50, 201, 206
diuretics 219, 220
domperidone 214
doxorubicin, pegylated 133
dry mouth 215
dysgerminoma 110, 118, 197–8
dyspnoea 220–1

embryonal carcinoma 199
endodermal sinus tumours 110, 198–9
endometrial cancer 145–52
   chemotherapy 103–4, 109, 111, 150
   complications of advanced disease
     233–4
   diagnosis/work-up 62–3, 145, 146–8
   epidemiology 3–6
   follow-up 151
   imaging 62–3, 146, 147–8
   multidisciplinary teams in 151–2
   palliative therapy 151
   pathology 20–2, 145–6
   radiotherapy 63, 99, 149–50
   recurrence 63, 99, 148, 149
   staging 147, 247

surgery 74–7, 85, 148–9, 234
endometrial hyperplasia 5–6, 21–2, 145
endometrial stromal tumours 22, 31, 204, 251
endometriosis 9, 26
EORTC trial 71, 107, 129, 130
epidemiology 1–11, 36, 38
  cervical cancer 1–3, 155
  endometrial cancer 3–6
  fallopian tube cancer 193
  GTD 189, 190
  ovarian cancer
    epithelial 1, 6–9, 115, 137
    nonepithelial 196, 197, 198
  vaginal cancer 201
  vulval cancer 9–10, 170
estrogen, as a risk factor 3, 4–5, 145
estrogen-secreting tumours 5, 118, 200
etoposide 107, 110, 118, 193, 198
exenteration, pelvic 62, 73, 84, 126–7, 162–3, 164

fallopian tube cancer 193–6, 254
febrile neutropenia 242
Fellow's vein 236
fentanyl 213
fertility, retention of 70, 110, 118, 127, 160–1
fibroids (leiomyoma) 24, 146
FIGO staging 19, 125, 177, 245–54
fistulae 221–3, 233, 238, 243
fluid imbalance 240–1
  see also ascites
5-fluorouracil 109
follow-up protocols
  cervical cancer 163–4
  endometrial cancer 151
  GTD 192, 193
  ovarian cancer 57–8, 136
frozen sections 16
fungating tumours 223–4

gastrointestinal complications
  advanced disease 58, 213–17, 225, 231–2
  chemotherapy 105, 242
  opioids 213
  radiotherapy 98, 243
  surgery 70, 231, 234, 238–9, 240

gemcitabine 133
genetics
  mutations found in various cancers 21, 26, 32
  risk factors 2–3, 7, 137–8
genital warts 170
germ-cell tumours 70, 110, 118, 196–9, 206
gestational trophoblastic disease (GTD) 64, 109–10, 111, 189–93, 252–3
granisetron 214, 242
granulosa cell tumours 5, 110, 118, 200
GROINSV trials 175, 176, 180
GTD see gestational trophoblastic disease

haemorrhage
  in advanced disease 224, 233, 233–4
  intra- and postoperative 75, 91, 235–6, 239–40
  see also bleeding
haloperidol 214, 215, 225
hCG (human chorionic gonadotrophin) 192
heparin 233, 235
hereditary non-polyposis colorectal cancer (HNPCC) 7, 137, 138
hernias, incisional 241–2
herpes simplex virus (HSV) 10
hormonal therapy for cancer 32, 107, 109, 133, 150–1
hormone replacement therapy (HRT)
  post-treatment 150–1, 164
  as a risk factor 5, 8
human chorionic gonadotrophin (hCG) 192
human leucocyte antigens (HLA) 2–3
human papillomavirus (HPV) 2, 9, 37–40
hydatidiform mole 189, 190–1, 192, 252
hyoscine butylbromide 215, 225
hypercalcaemia of malignancy 224
hypertension 5
hysterectomy
  cervical cancer/CIN 46, 73–4, 161
  complications 74, 75, 235–8, 239
  GTD 193
  ovarian cancer 124
  techniques 86–8
  uterine cancer 74, 85, 148, 205, 234
  VAIN and 50

hysteroscopy 147

ICON trials 106, 131, 133, 134
ifosfamide 108
imaging 53–65
  ascites 218
  bowel obstruction 58, 232
  cervical cancer 58–62, 158, 159
  endometrial cancer 62–3, 146, 147–8
  GTD 64
  ovarian cancer 53–8, 120, 122, 135–6
  uterine sarcoma 63–4
  vulval cancer 65, 175
immunisation 38–9
immunohistochemistry 29–33
immunosuppressed patients 38
incidence 1–2, 3, 6, 9, 170
infections 234, 240, 242
infertility treatment 8
inguinal lymph nodes 78, 174–6, 178–9,
    180, 181
intraperitoneal chemotherapy 132

kidney failure 233

lactulose 216–17
laparoscopy 83–92
  complications 234, 238
  endometrial cancer 77, 85, 148
  ovarian cancer 85–6, 135
laparotomy
  cervical cancer 73
  compared with laparoscopy 87
  complications 68–9, 130, 231, 235–42
  endometrial cancer 74–6, 148
  fallopian tube cancer 195
  ovarian cancer 69–71, 122–30, 134–5
  see also exenteration, pelvic
laxatives 215, 216–17
leiomyoma (fibroids) 24, 146
leiomyosarcoma 24, 64, 204, 250
lichen sclerosus 10, 26, 169
LLETZ excision 46, 74, 160
lorazepam 221
lymph nodes
  in cervical cancer 60–1, 72, 73, 84, 160
  complications of lymphadenectomy
      235, 236, 239, 241
  dissection techniques 89–91

in endometrial cancer 62, 76, 85,
    148–9
  in ovarian cancer 127, 128
  in vulval cancer 65, 78, 172, 173,
    174–6, 178–9, 180–2, 184
lymphoedema 149, 184, 219–20, 241

magnetic resonance imaging (MRI) 54–5,
    59–60, 62, 63, 65, 147–8, 159
malodour 224, 233
melanoma, vulval 27–8, 31, 173
mesothelioma, peritoneal 28, 31
metastatic disease
  from the cervix 62, 165
  from the ovaries 55
  to the ovaries 30–1, 56, 121
  see also lymph nodes; recurrence
methotrexate 110
metoclopramide 214, 215, 225
micropapillary serous carcinoma 25, 150
midazolam 224, 225
minimum deviation adenocarcinoma 20
mixed germ-cell tumours 199
mixed müllerian tumours of the uterus
    (carcinosarcoma) 22, 63, 146,
    204, 251
molar pregnancy see gestational
    trophoblastic disease
morphine 213, 215, 220, 223, 225
mortality rates 1, 2, 3, 6, 9
MRI see magnetic resonance imaging
mucinous tumours 25–6, 28–9
multidisciplinary teams 122, 151–2, 155,
    163, 209–10

nausea 213–14, 225, 242
neoadjuvant chemotherapy 71, 106, 107,
    109, 130
neoadjuvant radiotherapy 178, 182–3
nerve injuries, intraoperative 239
neuropathic pain 212, 223
neutropenia 105, 242
non-steroidal anti-inflammatory drugs
    (NSAIDs) 212
nulliparity 4, 7
nurse specialists 122, 210

obesity 4, 85, 234
obturator nerve 89, 239

octreotide 215
oncogenesis 6, 36, 39–40
ondansetron 214, 242
oophorectomy
  in ovarian cancer 124, 127, 197–8,
        199, 200, 201
  prophylactic 7, 138
  in uterine cancer 148, 205
opioids 211, 213, 215, 220, 223, 225
oral contraceptives 3, 4, 8
ovarian cancer (*epithelial unless indicated
        otherwise*) 115–39
  borderline tumours 25, 117
  chemotherapy 57, 71, 106–7, 111,
        130–4, 135–6
    nonepithelial tumours 110, 118,
        198, 199, 200
  complications of advanced disease 58,
        215, 218, 229–32
  diagnosis/work-up 30–1, 53–7, 85–6,
        119–22, 123
    nonepithelial tumours 197, 200
  epidemiology 1, 6–9, 115, 137
    nonepithelial tumours 196, 197, 198
  familial disease 137–8
  follow-up 57–8, 136
  germ-cell tumours 70, 110, 118,
        196–9, 206
  imaging 53–8, 120, 122, 135–6
  metastatic from other sites 30–1, 56,
        121
  monitoring therapy 57, 135–6
  multidisciplinary teams in 122
  paediatric 199, 206
  pathology 23–6, 116–18
  prognosis 118–19
  prophylaxis 7, 8, 138
  radiotherapy 100, 135
  recurrence 57–8, 71, 107, 132–5
  screening 7, 138–9
  sex-cord stromal tumours 5, 110, 118,
        199–201
  staging 86, 123, 125, 248
  surgery 56, 69–71, 85–6, 122–30, 134,
        135, 238–9, 240–1
    nonepithelial tumours 118, 197–8,
        199, 200, 201
ovarian cysts 8, 54, 55, 123, 124, 229

paclitaxel 106, 109, 131, 133, 195
paediatric tumours 199, 205–7
Paget's disease, extramammary 27, 31,
        169
pain relief 210–13, 215, 223, 225, 233
palliative care 209–26
  ascites 58, 217–19, 230–1
  breathlessness 220–1
  cervical cancer 165, 232
  chemotherapy 104, 107, 165
  emergencies 224, 230–4
  endometrial cancer 151
  fistulae 221–3, 233
  fungating tumours 223–4
  gastrointestinal symptoms 70, 213–17,
        225, 231–2
  haemorrhage 224, 233, 233–4
  lymphoedema 219–20
  ovarian cancer 58, 107, 135, 231, 232
  pain relief 210–13, 215, 223, 225, 233
  radiotherapy 100, 135, 165
  surgical 68, 78–9
  terminal phase 226, 233
Papanicolaou smear tests 40–2, 156
papillary serous tumours 25, 150
para-aortic lymph nodes 84, 85, 90–1,
        148–9, 239
paracentesis 58, 218–19, 231
paralytic ileus 232, 240
parametrium 60
parity, as a risk factor 4, 7
pathology 15–33
  cervical 16–20, 32, 35–6, 47
  endometrial 20–2, 145–6
  GTD 189–90
  immunohistochemistry 29–33
  ovarian 23–6, 116–18
  peritoneal 28–9, 31, 117
  specimen handling 15–16, 29
  uterine wall 22–3, 31, 146
  vulval 26–8, 31, 47–8, 169, 173
pelvic lymph nodes 60–1, 72, 73, 84, 160
  in cervical cancer 60–1, 72, 73, 84, 160
  dissection 89–90, 236, 239
  in endometrial cancer 62, 76, 85,
        148–9
  in vulval cancer 179
peritoneal pathology 28–9, 31, 117
PET *see* positron emission tomography

placental site trophoblastic tumours 190
pleural effusions 55
polycystic ovary syndrome 4
polyembryoma 199
positron emission tomography (PET) 58, 60–1, 62
postcoital bleeding 156
postmenopausal bleeding 4, 145, 146, 200
postoperative complications 69, 75, 130, 184, 231, 239–42
precocious pseudopuberty 199, 200
progestogens
  prophylactic 8
  therapeutic 109, 150
prognosis 32–3, 118–19
prophylaxis
  cervical cancer 38–9
  GTD 192
  ovarian cancer 7, 8, 138
psychological problems 42, 122

radical hysterectomy 73–4, 75, 86–8, 161, 238, 239
radiotherapy 95–101
  cervical cancer 61–2, 97, 98–9, 161–2, 165
  complications 62, 97–8, 150, 161, 243
  endometrial cancer 63, 99, 149–50
  fallopian tube cancer 195
  neoadjuvant 178, 182–3
  ovarian cancer 100, 135
  planning 61, 63, 96
  vaginal cancer 203
  vulval cancer 100, 178, 179–83
  see also chemoradiation
raloxifene 5
reconstructive surgery 68, 78, 183, 184
rectovaginal fistula 222, 233
rectum, radiotherapy and 96, 97
recurrence (relapse)
  cervical cancer 62, 73, 108, 164–5
  endometrial cancer 63, 99, 148, 149
  ovarian cancer 57–8, 71, 107, 132–5
  VIN 49
  vulval cancer 78–9, 183–4, 223
referral 120–1, 146, 152, 155–6, 157
renal failure 233
request forms for biopsy specimens 15–16

risk factors
  cervical cancer 2–3, 36
  endometrial cancer 4–6, 145
  GTD 190
  ovarian cancer 7–9, 137–8
  vaginal cancer 201
risk of malignancy index (RMI) 53–4, 85, 120

sarcoma
  cervical (sarcoma botryoides) 206
  fallopian tube 196
  uterine 22–3, 31, 63–4, 146, 204–5, 250–1
Schiller's test 45
screening
  for cervical cancer 40–6, 156
  for ovarian cancer 7, 138–9
second-look surgery 71, 128
sentinel lymph nodes 78, 84, 172, 175–6, 180, 184
serous carcinoma (ovarian) 25, 26, 31
Sertoli–Leydig tumours 200–1
sex-cord stromal tumours 5, 110, 118, 199–201
side effects see complications of treatment
smear tests 40–2, 156
smoking 3, 9, 10
spinal cord compression 224
squamous cell cancer 19, 27
  see also cervical cancer; vulval cancer
staging 32, 67–8
  cervical cancer 19, 71–2, 158–9, 246
  endometrial cancer 147, 247
  fallopian tube cancer 193, 254
  GTD 190, 252–3
  ovarian cancer 86, 123, 125, 248
  uterine sarcoma 250–1
  vaginal cancer 201–2, 254
  vulval cancer 176–7, 249
stratified mucinous intraepithelial lesion (SMILE) 18–19
surgery 67–80, 83–92
  complications 68–9, 70, 74, 75, 91, 130, 184, 203, 231, 234–42
  see also individual operative procedures and cancer sites
survival rates
  cervical cancer 1, 73

fallopian tube sarcoma 196
ovarian cancer 1, 6, 198
uterine cancer 1, 76, 205
vaginal cancer 204
vulval cancer 174
syringe drivers 225

talcum powder use 8
tamoxifen
  as a risk factor 5, 145
  therapy 107, 150
teratoma 110, 198
terminal phase 226, 233
thecoma 5, 200
thrombosis 233, 234, 240
topotecan 108, 133, 165
torsion of adnexal masses 229, 230
trachelectomy 59, 73, 74, 160
tranexamic acid 224, 233
transitional-cell carcinoma 201
tumour markers
  fallopian tube cancer 194
  granulosa cell tumours 200
  GTD 190, 192
  ovarian epithelial cancer 85, 120, 121,
    135, 136
  ovarian germ-cell tumours 197

ultrasound
  abdominal (for ascites) 218
  Doppler 64
  transvaginal 53–4, 62, 120, 146
ureteric injuries 75, 236–8
ureterovaginal fistula 238
urinary tract complications
  in advanced disease 58, 221–3, 233
  of radiotherapy 97, 98, 243
  of surgery 75, 236–8, 239
uterine artery 88, 236
uterine cancer 1
  endometrial see endometrial cancer
  mixed 22, 63, 146, 204, 251
  paediatric 206
  sarcoma 22–3, 31, 63–4, 146, 204–5,
    250–1

vaccination 38–9
vaginal cancer 65, 100, 201–4, 206–7, 254
vaginal hysterectomy 74, 87

vaginal intraepithelial neoplasia (VAIN)
    49–50, 163, 201
venous injuries, intraoperative 234, 235–6
venous thromboembolism 233, 234, 240
verrucous carcinoma (vulval) 27
vesicovaginal fistula 221, 233
VIN (vulval intraepithelial neoplasia)
    9–10, 26–7, 47–9, 169–70
virilisation 200, 201
vomiting 213–14, 225, 240, 242
vulval cancer 169–85
  chemoradiation 100, 109, 111, 182
  diagnosis/work-up 77, 170–6
  epidemiology 9–10, 170
  imaging 65, 175
  paediatric 207
  pathology 26–8, 31, 47–8, 169, 173
  radiotherapy 100, 178, 179–83
  recurrence 78–9, 183–4, 223
  staging 176–7, 249
  surgery 77–8, 177–9, 182–3, 184
vulval intraepithelial neoplasia (VIN)
    9–10, 26–7, 47–9, 169–70

wound dressings 224, 240